Belly Dancing

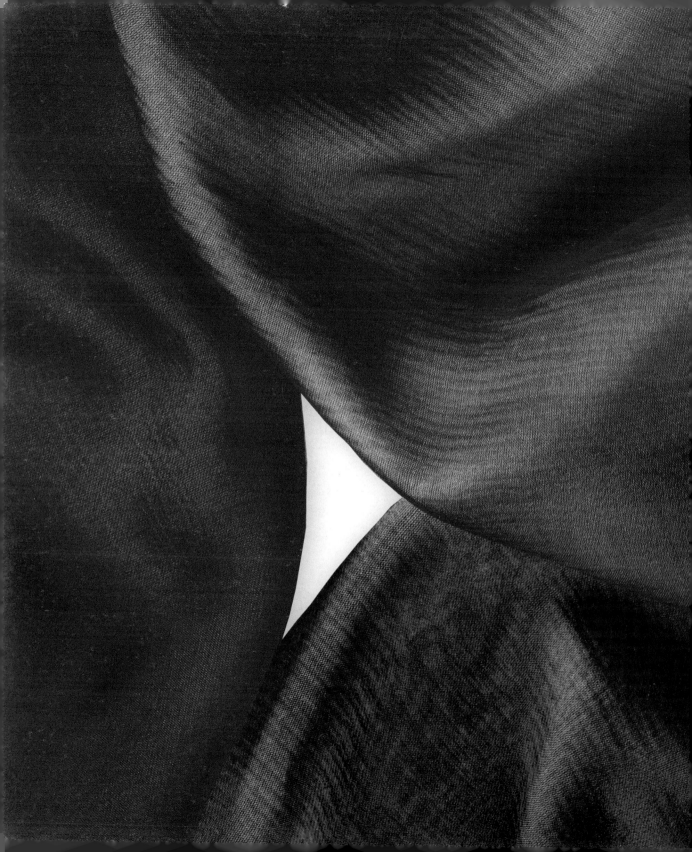

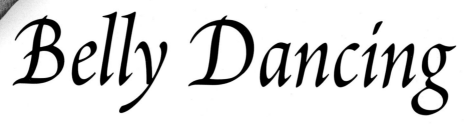

Belly Dancing

The Sensual Art of
Energy and Spirit

Pina Coluccia
Anette Paffrath
Jean Pütz

Park Street Press
Rochester, Vermont

Park Street Press
One Park Street
Rochester, Vermont 05767
www.InnerTraditions.com

Park Street Press is a division of Inner Traditions International

Originally published in Germany under the title *Bauchtanz* by Egmont vgs
  verlagsgesellschaft Köln
First U.S. edition published in 2005 by Park Street Press

Library of Congress Cataloging-in-Publication Data
Coluccia, Pina.
  [Bauchtanz. English]
  Belly dancing : the sensual art of energy and spirit / Pina Coluccia, Anette Paffrath, and
Jean Pütz.—1st U.S. ed.
    p. cm. 3339 4833 8/05
  Summary: "A comprehensive guide to the art of belly dancing"—Provided by
publisher.
  ISBN 1-59477-021-2
  1. Belly dance. I. Paffrath, Anette. II. Pütz, Jean. III. Title.
  GV1798.5.C6513 2005
  793.3—dc22
                              2004025005

Printed and bound in Italy

10 9 8 7 6 5 4 3 2 1

This book was typeset in Frutiger with Poetica Chancery as the display typeface

Photographs on pages 81 and 107 by Larry Gee

I dedicate this book to all women
who will dance their way to energy and beauty.
And I am grateful that the dance has brought us,
Pina and Jean, together in a partnership of love,
which has gifted us with our wonderful young son.

J. P.

Contents

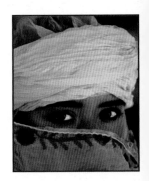

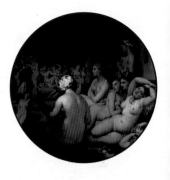

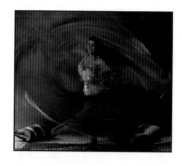

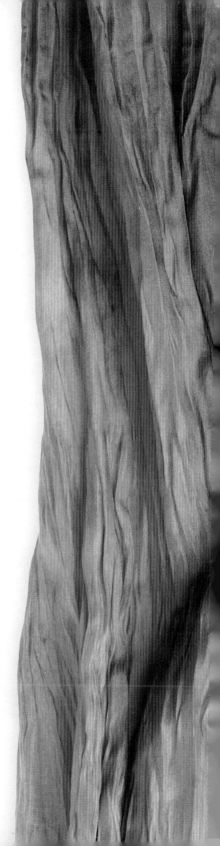

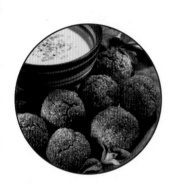

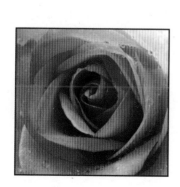

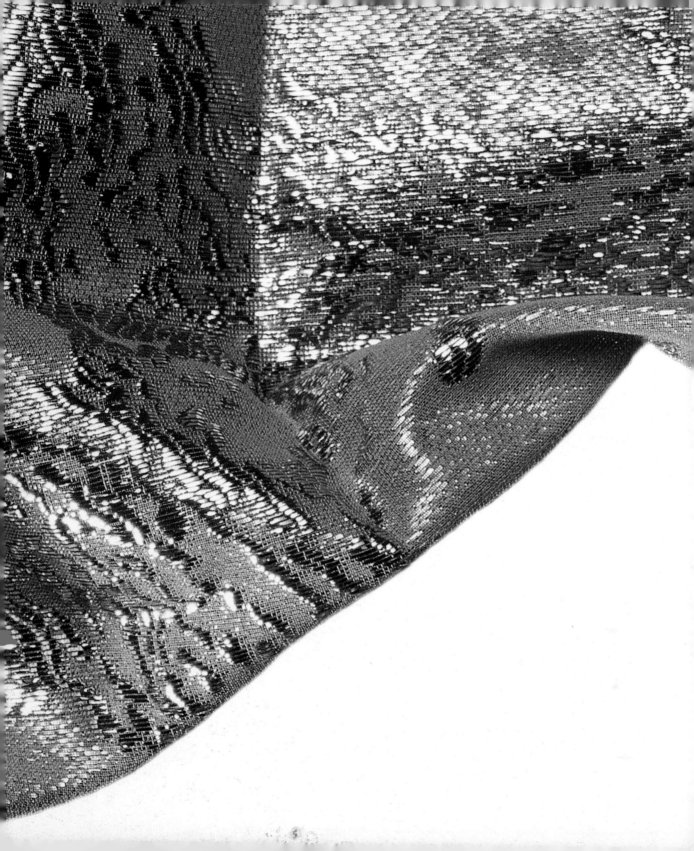

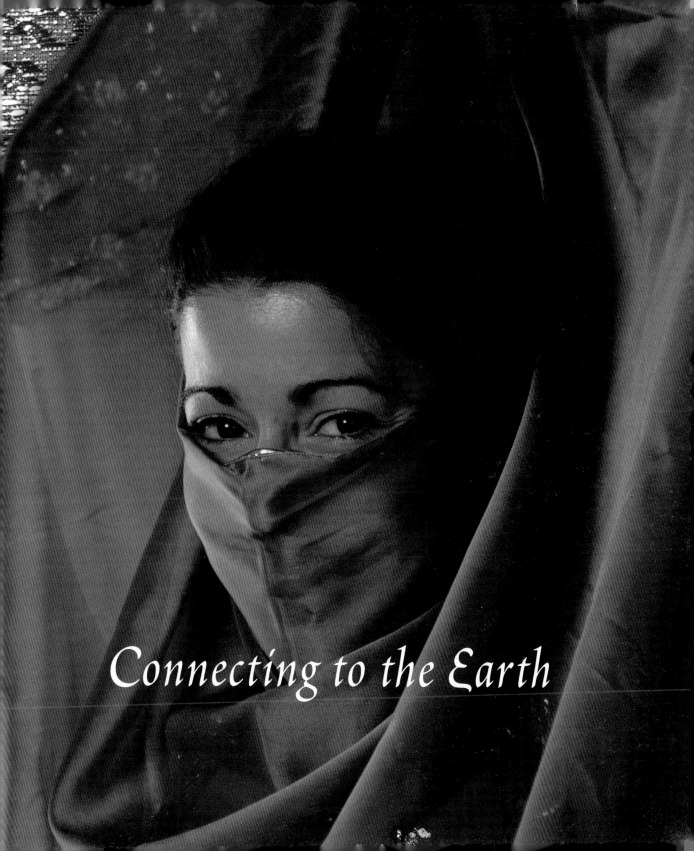

Connecting to the Earth

*G*racefully shaking her hips, the veiled dancer moves across the floor. She sways to the drumbeats, sensually gesturing with her arms toward the audience. As the tempo of the music quickens, she shakes her hips faster and faster, shimmying her entire body.

Performing what has become known as "belly dance," the dancer has tapped into the deep wisdom of her feminine essence. With belly (Oriental) dance a woman can discover her body, and through the dance she can express her character and her soul, embodying the myriad facets of femininity. A woman may want to proclaim her wholeness and independence, dancing to show that she feels full and powerful within the world. She may want to dance in celebration of beauty and love that she feels inside. She may dance to celebrate motherhood and the power that she has to love, care for, and protect her children. She could dance to celebrate transitions in life stages from maiden to mother to crone.

Belly dance allows women to connect with their inner thoughts and feelings and identities and learn to express these things through movement. To experience these different expressions of femininity, to live different female roles in the dance, has therapeutic value. Women can reclaim their identities, defining themselves in terms of qualities they admire in the Goddess or in themselves; reconnecting with an inner spiritual core gives extra energy and a sense of power. Understanding the self and connecting the identity to the body allows for a holistic understanding of identity, one based both in emotional and physical realms. Even as a show dance, belly dance can free a woman to experience her beauty and eroticism. In learning the dance, a woman unlocks an energy and power from deep inside herself.

The dancer Yemaya notes that the dancer communicates her self-understanding to the audience when she performs. Yemaya says that the creative energy of the dance transforms the dancer, allowing her to reimagine

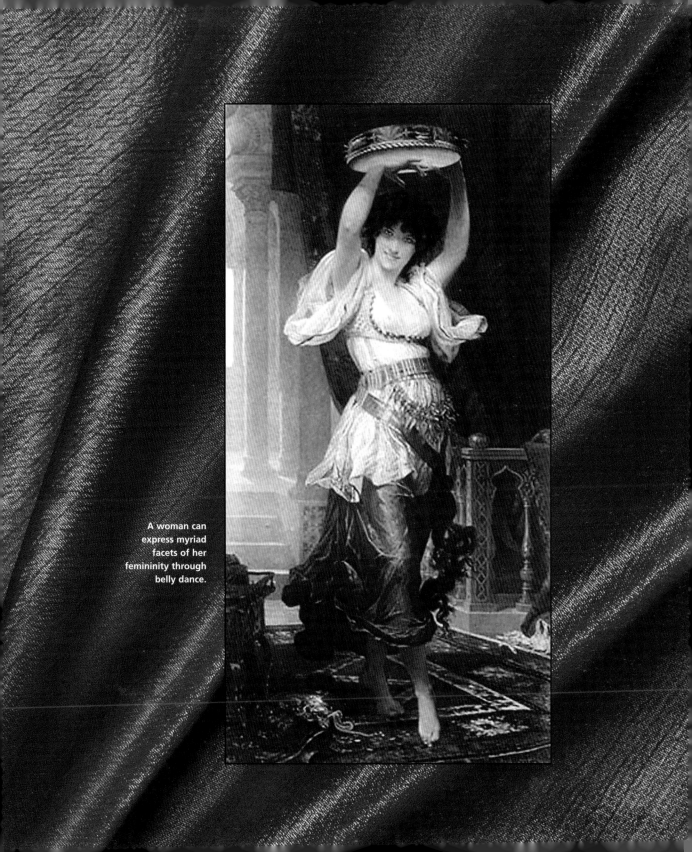

A woman can express myriad facets of her femininity through belly dance.

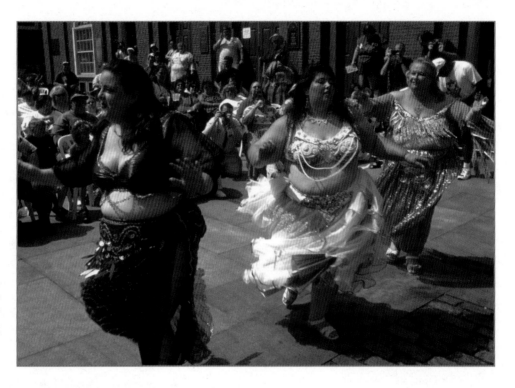

herself and free herself from the constricts of her own mind. Energetic women might discover an affinity for shimmies during drum rolls, embodying the role of a magician who entrances people with her dance. Dancing with a veil and moving her arms, a woman can express elegance and tenderness. She can play the role of Scheherazade, who is young, smart, mysterious, and playful. Women who usually think of themselves as lethargic and slow might discover their playfulness and ease of movement, unlocking the maiden within.

A playful dancer might think of herself as the maiden in the maidenmother-crone triple-goddess typology. The maiden, confident in herself, runs across the landscape, playing and laughing. Sure of herself, she laughs and dances, carefree and beautiful. She knows only the beauty and reliability of her body and the happiness of life. We will see an example of the maiden goddess when we look at Artemis, the celibate hunter and Great Mother.

In ancient times, dancing was a form of communication between the human corporeal realm and the ethereal spirit realm. Dancing loosened the body, allowing the vital energies to flow more freely within and outside of the body. By dancing, women opened their vital energy centers to receive

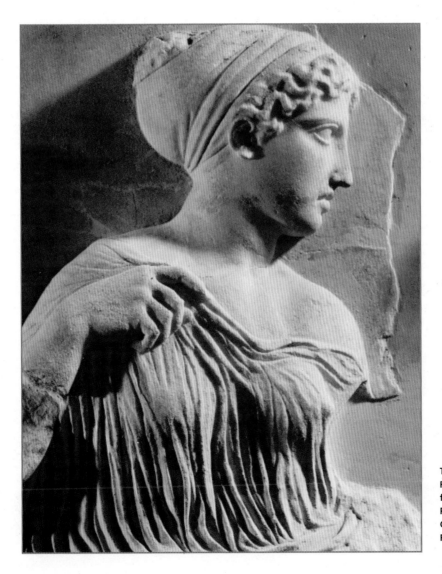

The goddess Artemis. Relief (ca. 440–432 B.C.E.) from the east frieze of the Parthenon, Athens, Greece. Erich Lessing/Art Resource, NY.

divine wisdom and to give wisdom to others. In dancing, a woman can reconnect with that power and free her soul once more. Dancing allows us to forget our inhibitions and daily responsibilities. By moving to the beat, we embrace the moment and allow ourselves to experience deeply. This experience gives us power because it connects us with deeper truths and wisdoms that we carry within our souls. Living fully and truly experiencing the dance allows for revitalization of our inner understandings and makes us feel more complete.

A swirl of color and form. Gypsy Caravan performs at Edgefield Oktoberfest 2003, Troutdale, Oregon. Photograph by Larry Gee.

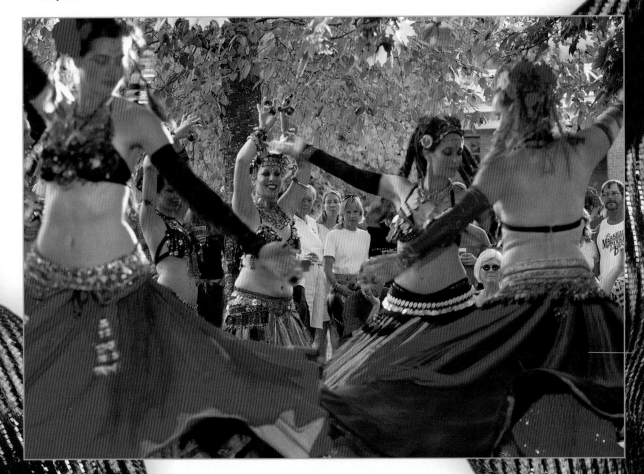

Flowing Energy in a Grounded Body

In Arabic the belly dance is called *raqs sharqi,* which translates as "Oriental dance." The belly dance is actually a dance that encompasses all body parts, from the soles of the feet to the tips of the hairs. Most movements originate from the body's center. The spinal cord is the steady axis around which the pelvis and chest rotate. The spine remains steady during the circling of the head; the head remains upright. During the movement commonly known as "the shimmy," the pelvis or chest vibrate. These vibrations loosen the shoulder and pelvic girdles.

Belly dance is not a room-filling dance. Movements spread in rhythmic waves across the body—the body itself becomes the space for the dance, and the dancer dances with and within her own body. This is entirely different from such dance forms as classical ballet, in which the dancer moves across the room through jumps and turns, often with a partner. The ballet dancer appears to float or fly, attempting to create the illusion of weightlessness.

In contrast, belly dance is a very grounded dance. The basic position from which movements originate connects the dancer with the earth. Belly dance gets its beauty not from strength but from the dancer's ability to play selectively with her muscles. This selective muscular engagement is why shimmies appear so easy and effortless when performed by experienced dancers.

Belly dancing requires the dancer to ground herself within her body, to connect with the earth and inhabit her space. Rather than shunning and hiding her feminine form and the creative, mothering power that her body represents, the woman who wants to belly dance must embrace her body and its movements. Belly dancing, for many women, offers a way of speaking back to a culture that demands that a female body be thin and that women remain small and quiet at the edges of culture. Belly dancers enter a room with presence, proud of what their bodies can do and what they communicate. By learning how to belly dance, women can understand

7

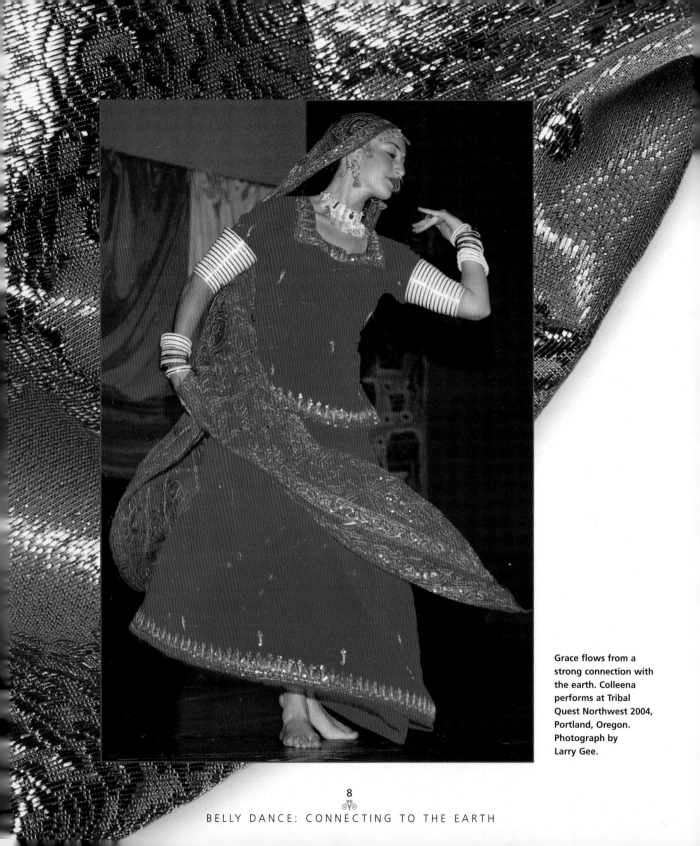

Grace flows from a strong connection with the earth. Colleena performs at Tribal Quest Northwest 2004, Portland, Oregon. Photograph by Larry Gee.

how to better love themselves and express themselves through movement. Furthermore, dancers can communicate their transformations to their audience and allow the audience to be transformed as well.

To understand the dance we will begin by considering the possible origins of belly dance. While there is certainly no consensus about where and why belly dance began, surveying the origin myths illustrates how women have developed their own stories to inspire their practice of this ancient art form.

The Origins of Belly Dancing

To illustrate the ambiguous history of belly dancing, we will begin by looking at the terminology surrounding the dance. The name "belly dance" is used mostly in North America and Europe. Some scholars attribute the term to the French *danse du ventre* (literally: "dance of the stomach"), an epithet first used to disparage a Middle Eastern dance performance at the 1893 World's Fair in Chicago. Others claim that "belly dance" is borrowed from the Arabic word *beledi,* meaning "country" and indicating the indigenous nature of the belly dance, a dance that changes in different communities and expresses communal identities and beliefs. Regardless of how the term emerged, "belly dance" refers to a modern Middle Eastern dance style that is popular today, an improvisation on and innovation of ancient techniques.

Some dancers and authors prefer to call the dance "Oriental dance," referring to dances of the East, from Turkey to China and Japan. Still other scholars further break down the geographic origins of the dance, referring to their work as "Middle Eastern" and "Near Eastern" dance. Finally, there is the growing "American (or urban) tribal" style, a manner of dancing in which a number of dancers work together as a choreographed group blending styles from many different countries.

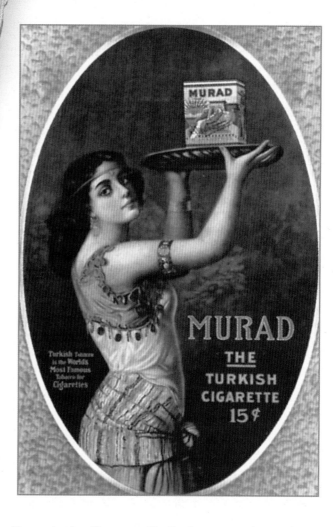

After the 1893 World's Fair, "Orientalist" images began appearing in popular culture.

In this book, we will use the familiar term "belly dance" to discuss both the ancient Eastern styles of dance and the more modern traditions that have grown from the older styles. However, it is important to know that there are many variations of belly dance and the dance does change from community to community.

Belly dance has a richly mythologized past from which dancers can draw energy, passion, and inspiration. One origin story connects the development and spread of belly dance to the migration of the Roma (Gypsies) from the Indian subcontinent in the eleventh century. Traveling across Europe, Asia, and the Middle East, these wanderers introduced their style of dancing to the indigenous traditions extant in the societies that they encountered. In places where societies were sex-segregated, men and women developed separate dances that were performed within the group.

If a woman considers herself a traveler or wanderer, perhaps this origin story would appeal to her. She can think of herself as a wandering Roma,

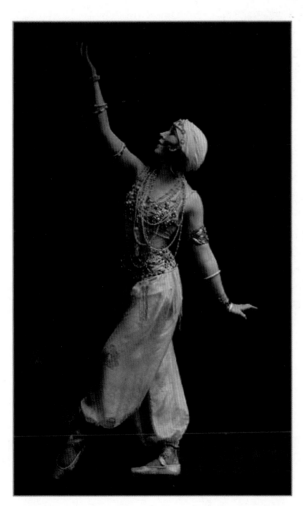

An image from the past: a postcard titled "Danze d'oriente."

BELLY DANCE: CONNECTING TO THE EARTH

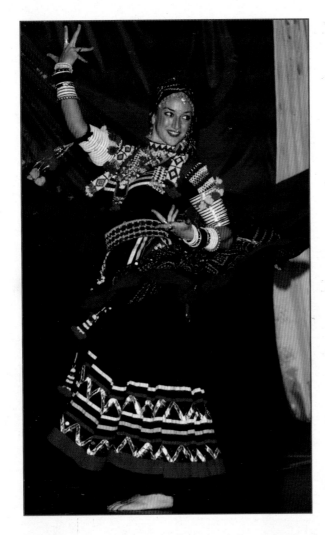

bringing new dance and music to share with other communities. She teaches others how to communicate with the divine using their bodies.

Dance played a prominent role in both the royal and lay societies of ancient Egypt. Dancing was an important component in Egyptian worship of the gods and goddesses and in the mythology of the gods and goddesses themselves. Ancient Egyptians believed that they were given dance by the goddesses Hathor and Isis; in turn, humans used dance to beseech these great goddesses for fertility.

Dance was connected to ancient Egyptian astrology, with priests mimicking the movement of the planets through the movement of their bodies. It has been suggested that astrology in ancient Egypt was a part of the religious beliefs and that priests could use their knowledge of the planets to see into the future. By mimicking the movements of the planets in their dances, perhaps the priests were worshipping these celestial instruments. In ancient Egyptian society, astrological energies were the major deciding factors about when planting would begin; they also determined which gods should be worshipped when and dictated the activities of the populace on different

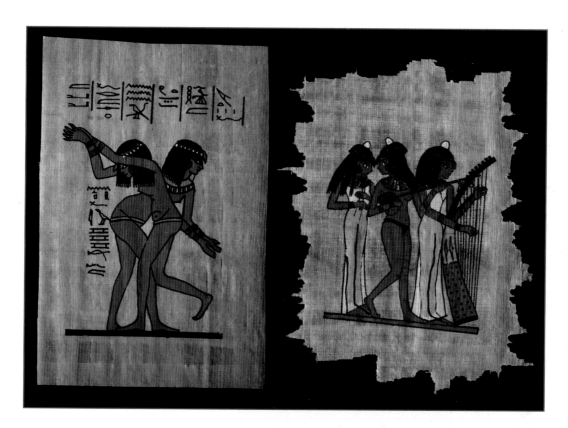

days. Astrology was taken extremely seriously, and the priests, as astrologoers, therefore had a very important social role. They not only acted as representatives of the pharaoh but they also created the astrological calendar that dictated the rhythm of social life.

Priests mimicking the orbit of the planets through dance therefore suggests worship of the planets or at the very least an acknowledgment of the power of the planets to provide knowledge of the future. In ancient Egypt, dances were used as worship, at harvest, to celebrate specific religious festivals, and at funerals.

Ancient Egyptians also used dance to communicate outside the religious realm. Some scholars suggest that dance gained such an important

Salome and the Dance of the Seven Veils

In the Bible, no name is given to the woman who dances for Herod and then demands the head of John the Baptist. John the Baptist reprimanded King Herod because of his unseemly living with his sister-in-law Herodias, Salome's mother. Herod has John the Baptist incarcerated because of his outspokenness. During a dinner, Salome, the daughter of Herod's lover, dances so appealingly that Herod grants her the fulfillment of any wish. At the insistence of her adulterous mother, Salome asks for John the Baptist's head, which is served to her on a platter handed to her by Herod (Matthew 14:11).

The description of this incident in the Bible makes it clear that Herodias took the chance to do away with the man who was harming her reputation. It was she who desired the death of John the Baptist. Viewed in this light, Salome was being used by her mother to exert her power. Indeed, other sources suggest that Salome was a companion of John the Baptist. The fact that Salome probably supported his teachings might have been one more reason for her mother to have him disposed.

Salome can be seen as a woman who uses her body and her erotic power as a means to an end. This interpretation serves to depict female attraction and Eros as destructive and dangerous.

However, Salome could also have been a priestess, a woman in the service of the goddess. Her recasting in the Bible as an evil seductress who martyrs John the Baptist could represent a biblical subjugation of the older goddess-worshipping tradition. In the Sumerian tradition, there is the story of Ishtar/Inanna's descent into the underworld to rescue Tammuz who has been trapped. At each of the seven gates Ishtar removes a garment, symbols of her power, to experience death, enter the underworld, and save Tammuz. This story could have been recast in early Christian tradition in the story of Salome as a dance of seduction, rather than as a journey of a powerful goddess to rescue her lover. In other words, Salome the priestess could have become Salome the evil seductress in the biblical retelling of the story to present the superiority of the male-dominated Christian tradition over the female-dominated goddess tradition.

Another version of the story tells of Ishtar removing valuable jewelry and other material goods and giving them away at the seven gates of the underworld. Regardless, it is the goddess Ishtar's sacred love and sacrifice that helps Tammuz to be reincarnated; the goddess of fertility was thus also considered the goddess of resurrection. The great mother could both create and destroy, bringing the killing infertile season with her grief for Tammuz yet also resurrecting him by bringing him back from the dead and allowing plants to grow again. People of those times buried their dead in stomach-shaped containers (called *pitus*), in the fetal position. This container they gave to the earth. In this goddess they saw the Earth Mother, who ensures that new life comes from the earth.

Mary as Virginal Goddess

According to standard theological historical science, parts of Sumerian mythos were incorporated into the Bible as well. The story of Mary and Jesus show parallels to Sumerian mythos, even though the message of the Bible is very different. The virgin goddess corresponds to the Virgin Mary. Jesus, the savior who is resurrected after his death, is a sign of reincarnation and gives people hope. We can also read Mary as the mother goddess who, like Ishtar, births her son only to give him up to death. Jesus, like Tammuz, descends to the underworld and then is reborn. Although biblical theology strips Mary of her centrality and sexuality, she still resembles the mother goddess and her life-giving powers.

With the annual death of Tammuz and the descent of Ishtar, the moon's power would wane and no water would come to nourish the crops. As long as the goddess was in the underworld, "the fields would be barren, animals no longer mate, and the man no longer sleeps with the woman." Only with the ascent of Tammuz and Ishtar would a new growth cycle begin. So, like Kali in the Indian tradition, the Mesopotamian Ishtar has both the power to create and the power to destroy. Under her different names, Ishtar was the most important goddess of the ancient Near East. She existed as the ultimate mother, the goddess who reigned over all. Even

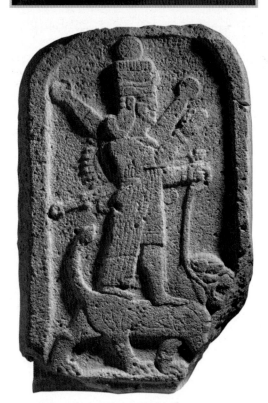

Ishtar, goddess of love, standing on her iconographic animal, the lion. Assyrian, 8th century B.C.E. Erich Lessing/Art Resource, NY.

though she had a husband, brother, and lover in the god Tammuz, it is Ishtar who controls the weather and the growing of the crops. Because of her love for Tammuz, Ishtar fearlessly descends into the underworld, rescuing him and bringing life back to earth. She uses her power to demonstrate her love for Tammuz and for humans and to save both.

Ishtar was also a powerful healer, a bringer of fertility, and a goddess of war and power. She oversaw all important human endeavors and was worshipped as the goddess who controlled the universe. In Babylonian scriptures such as the Gilgamesh, the ancient epic of the creation of the universe, Ishtar plays a central role. She is called "Light of the World, Leader of Hosts, Opener of the Womb, Righteous Judge, Lawgiver, Goddess of Goddesses, Bestower of Strength, Framer of all Decrees, Lady of Victory, Forgiver of Sins, Torch of Heaven and Earth."

Ishtar is a powerful archetype that can be used in inspiring a dance. She represents complete divinity within femininity, a goddess who is complete and powerful within her female form. She does not need a male consort; she chooses to love Tammuz and chooses to

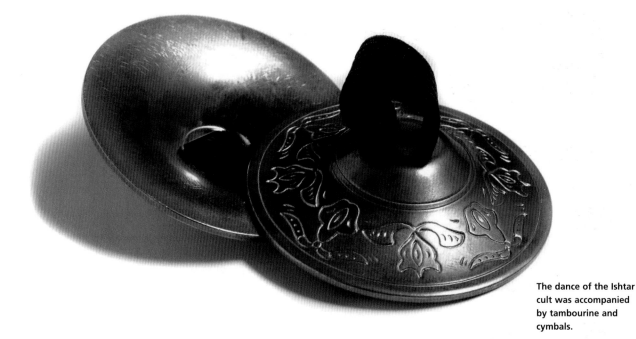

The dance of the Ishtar cult was accompanied by tambourine and cymbals.

live with him for six months of the year. Ishtar represents love and loss, creation and destruction, peace and war. Her power exists in all of us who choose to look for our completion within our own souls rather than looking to another to complete us.

Ishtar is the great mother, the goddess who looks over us all. She is the Queen of Heaven. When you dance as Ishtar, envision yourself as the Queen of Heaven, the goddess who seeks wholeness from within. Harness the energy of the dance to find the power of the universe within yourself. Ishtar uses her own resources and abilities to control the universe, to save Tammuz, and to help humans with disease and infertility. When you dance as Ishtar, you connect to this powerful legacy. Feel the spirit of Ishtar flow into your dance. Embrace her power and see how it can help you in your own life.

The connections between the goddess, dance, and fertility transcended ancient Mesopotamian culture and extended into Greek and Roman cultures through the goddesses Artemis and Aphrodite. The ancient Greek Artemis is best known as the celibate goddess of the hunt. However, under the names Kordax and Hegemone, Artemis also was the goddess of maiden dances and hymns. As a celibate goddess, she represented the maiden stage of a woman's life, the time before sexuality, fertility, and motherhood.

One myth says that immediately after her birth, Artemis, who was born on the island of Ortygia, helped her mother, Leto, cross the ocean to Delos to give birth to her twin brother, Apollo. From that moment onward, Artemis became the protector of women in childbirth and of young children. However, like Ishtar, Artemis embodies both the creative and destructive aspects of life. Although she protects women in labor, it is Artemis's arrows that take life from women who die in labor. And although she is a healing goddess, Artemis also brings such diseases as gout and leprosy. Perhaps her dual nature, like Ishtar's dual nature, illustrates Artemis's complete nature as the celibate goddess of the hunt. Like Ishtar, Artemis creates and destroys in her own image, without the assistance of a male consort. Indeed, there are many stories of Artemis punishing men who attempt to take her chastity. Her peaceful and wrathful sides illustrate the holistic nature of Artemis's image.

Artemis travels around the forest with her nymphs, protecting her sacred animals. She does not hestitate to punish those who harm her animals, in the same way that she defends her chastity and the chastity of her nymphs. Orion felt Artemis's wrath when he tried to take her honor; in one myth, Artemis conjured a scorpion that killed Orion and his dog. Orion and the scorpion became constellations in the sky, while Orion's dog can now be seen as Sirius, the dog star.

Artemis was worshipped in most Greek cities, especially Arcadia, Sparta, Laconia, Mount Taygetus, Elis, and the forested areas of Greece. In Asia

Minor (modern Turkey), particularly the city of Ephesus, Artemis was a major fertility deity, known as Cybele, a mother goddess. There was a major temple built in her honor. In Ephesus, a different form of Artemis developed. In the areas near modern Greece, Artemis was normally depicted as the huntress, standing with her bows and arrows. However, in Ephesus, in Asia Minor, where she was seen as a major great mother goddess (in the same vein as Ishtar), Artemis can been seen with breasts covering her torso. This form suggests Artemis's importance as a fertility goddess. Interestingly, this form of Artemis developed in the part of ancient Greece located in the Near East, closest to those regions where Ishtar gained prominence as the great mother goddess. Furthermore, it has been suggested that Artemis's temple was built in a region controlled by female warriors (Amazons). Perhaps there is some connection between the preeminence of Ishtar in the Middle East and the development

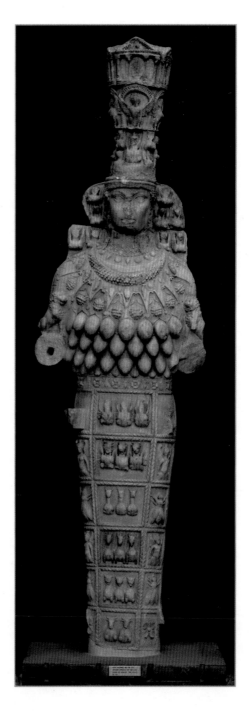

Grand Artemis, first half of the 2nd century C.E., Slecuk, Ephesus Archeological Museum.

of Artemis as a many-breasted fertility goddess and great mother in the Near East.

Artemis, like Ishtar, represents many different ways for women to act in the world. On one hand, she is a huntress, a powerful woman who challenges those men who attempt to take over her domain. On the other hand, she appears covered with many breasts, literally able to feed the world, and is the protector of mothers and young children. Artemis also was the goddess of maidens and young women. When young girls reached puberty, a time of change and tremendous female power, they were initiated into Artemis's cult. When these women decided to marry, they left their childhood toys along with some hair in front of the altar of Artemis to signify their transition from celibate maidens to fertile women. Artemis looks over women and protects them throughout their lives.

As in ancient Egypt, dance was an important method of worshipping deities in ancient Greece. Many different types of dance developed, such as circle dances around sacred objects, solemn dances and processions, and festival dancing. Artemis is one of the Greek deities honored through dance and festivals. As the great mother goddess, it is not inconceivable that belly dance was used to worship her, especially given Artemis's role as a fertility goddess and protector of children, virgins, and women in labor. Young girls, as they began the transition into puberty, would play games and perform rituals at the temple of Artemis as a way of marking this important transition and continuing to curry the favor of this powerful goddess.

Evoking Artemis as an archetype for dance, like using Ishtar, is a way of expressing fullness and completion in the self. Artemis is a powerful goddess who protects those who may be weak or hurt, such as young children, women in labor, animals, and in some myths, women who have been sexually assaulted. Dancing with Artemis could help to make you feel stronger and more empowered.

Perhaps if you protect others in your daily life, using Artemis as an archetype will help you to share your burden. Artemis dances for herself

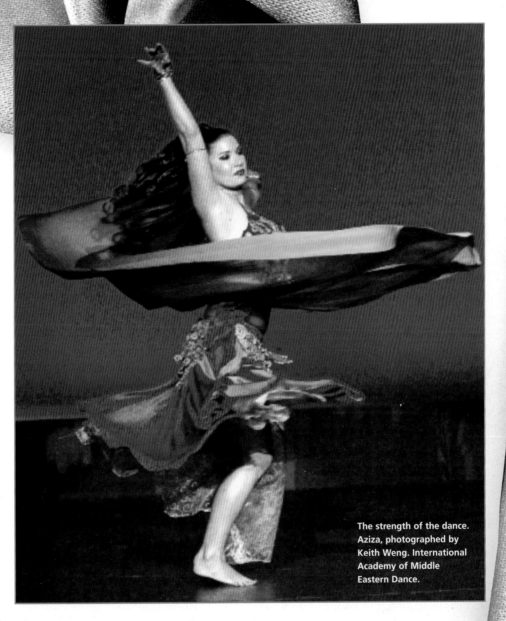

The strength of the dance. Aziza, photographed by Keith Weng. International Academy of Middle Eastern Dance.

and to show her strength for others. She is a strong, proud goddess who rejects those who would try to control her. She helps those around her through difficult times. She is an Amazon, a woman warrior, and her

BELLY DANCE: CONNECTING TO THE EARTH

ferocity protects while it intimidates. When you imagine yourself as Artemis in the dance, you invoke power, protection, pride, and wholeness.

The goddess Aphrodite, known as the Greek love goddess, also had roots in the ancient Middle East, descending from Astarte/Aschera, the great mother goddess of Syria. As ancient mother of the Romans, Aphrodite gave birth to Aeneas, the mythical founder of Rome. Under the name Venus she was the mother of the Venetians. She also carried the names Mari, Marina, and Stella Maris, all of which imply her power over the sea.

The goddess of fertility, birth, marriage, and sexuality, Aphrodite stands for sensual passion. The main place for the worshipping of Aphrodite was Paphos on the island of Cyprus. It was here that Aphrodite was said to have stepped out of the ocean fully formed. The beginning of her name, *aphros,* means "foam," indicating her formation in the ocean.

One of the major holy places of Aphrodite was the city Aphrodisias (the ruins of which are located near the village of Geyre in southwestern Turkey), which was once dedicated to the goddess Ishtar, the temple of Aphrodite being erected on the fundaments of an Ishtar temple. Up to the seventh century (and experiencing a brief revival in the eleventh century), the goddess was worshipped there as a patron of arts, sciences, crafts, and education.

Aphrodite had the power to make everyone—including deities—fall in love or become aroused. She had a belt that made its wearer irresistible. In the worshipping of Aphrodite we find the worship of female beauty, attraction, and sensuality. We also see the continuation of the Great Mother Goddess, the one who presides over the generative powers of the body.

Unlike Ishtar and Artemis, Aphrodite was an overtly sexual goddess. This goddess of beauty, love, and sexual desire and fulfillment oversees passion and desire in wedlock. As Artemis watches over women in the maiden

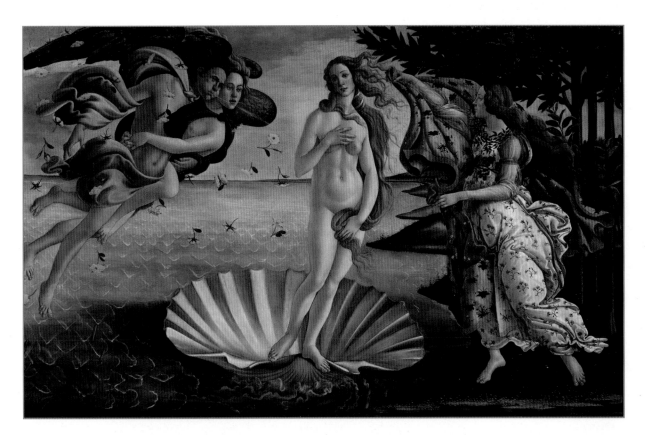

The Roman
goddess Venus is
equivalent to the
Greek goddess
Aphrodite. *The
Birth of Venus*,
Sandro Botticelli,
ca. 1485, Florence.

stage of life, Aphrodite protects women as mothers, women in marriages, and women in the throes of sexual passion. It has been suggested that Aphrodite is another form of Ishtar, brought to Greece by sea traders. She certainly fulfills the Great Mother role, the woman who watches over women within marriage. Unlike Ishtar and Artemis, Aphrodite had many lovers, including Zeus, Hermes, and Dionysus.

Aphrodite's priestesses worshipped her through having sex with men who came to honor the goddess. These women were not seen as prostitues, but as devotees performing an essential act of worship to the goddess of love and sexuality. In Aphrodite we see an acknowledgement of the importance of the body, of love and sexuality, especially female sexuality.

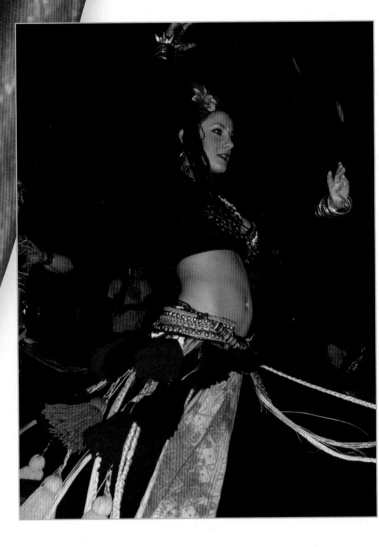

Sunny of
Barika
Bellydance,
2003.
Photograph
by Xian.

Rather than shaming the female body, worshippers of Aphrodite rejoiced in the power and enjoyment of sexuality.

In addition to sexual intercourse, dance was an important method of worshipping Aphrodite. After slaying the Minotaur, Theseus stopped on the island of Dinos (the birthplace of Artemis) to offer a sacrifice to Aphrodite, the goddess of love. This dance, called the *geranos*, involves mimicking Theseus's journey through the labyrinth using "serpentine" movements. These movements, originally done around the altar of Aphrodite, suggest a connection to worshipping the goddess through belly dance. Another dance connected to Aphrodite is *imeneos,* the dance of marriage. This dance is performed by the bride, her mother, and the other women at the wedding. It is fast, and like geranos, has many twisting motions. Again, we can see a connection between the flowing and turning motions of belly dance and these ancient dances of Aphrodite. Furthermore, archaelogical evidence shows dancers at the temple, dancing with arms and faces raised to the sky to honor the goddess. Women wearing beautiful clothing and jewelry are depicted in Aphrodite's temples, and some of these women danced to honor the goddess.

By using Aphrodite as an archetype, you can connect to the celebration of sexuality that she represents. More obviously than Ishtar and Artemis, Aphrodite represents female sensuality, the magic that occurs through sexual connection. Perhaps you will choose to dance more sensuously when you are dancing with Aphrodite. However, Aphrodite is also the goddess of beauty and of love, and it is important to remember that while sensuality is certainly full of beauty and love, love and beauty also exist separately from sexuality. When you connect to Aphrodite, you connect to the energy of love, and whether or not you choose to invoke sexuality with that love, you can still use the archetype of the beautiful foam-born Aphrodite to inspire your dance.

The Goddess and Sexuality

Worship of the divine feminine is becoming more widespread today. Although we lack historical knowledge of ancient goddess-worshipping and matrilineal societies, many men and women are attempting to reconnect with an idea of the Great Goddess, the divine feminine. In our quest

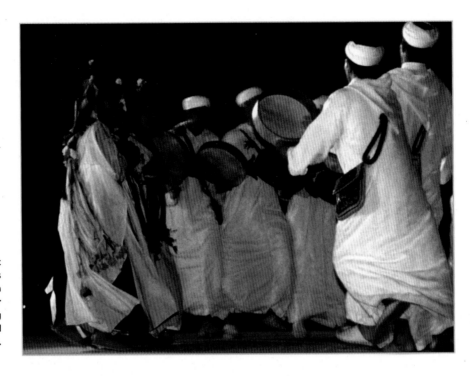

to discover the power of the goddess, we must connect with our bodies and our sexuality, because the goddess in many cultures was connected to sexuality and to the exclusively female act of birthing.

In all cultures in which the Great Goddess was celebrated, people believed that sexual desire and fertility were gifts from the goddess. Sexuality represented the will of life itself and was considered a creative energy through which new life arose.

According to this belief, the world was created from a wedding night, from an erotic encounter of ancient cosmic forces. It was not the love for a person that was considered holy, but love, the sexual connection itself. According to this belief, the willingness of women and men to give themselves to love and to present the goddess with their sexuality was thought to please the goddess and to give humans a plentiful harvest. Initiation rituals, held in honor of the goddess, celebrated the memory of the bridal night, the creation of the world. Men visited the temple to be initiated into the mysteries of the goddess through a sexual encounter with a priestess. Young women spent a period of time in the temple and served the goddess by offering their sexuality before they got married. We see these practices in the worship of both Artemis and Aphrodite. Before marriage, women served Artemis and her temple. Priestesses of Aphrodite united with men to more fully worship the goddess of love and sexuality.

In the Sumerian/Mesopotamian belief system, the priestesses of Ishtar were considered not only healers but also magicians, prophets, and visionaries. A woman's bodily fluids were regarded to have healing powers and

Men and Belly Dance

Men also have a history of performing belly dance. In ancient Egypt, men performed combat dances that showed their prowess as warriors and retold the history of the dynasty. Men were experts at the saber dance. Among the Pygmies, men carry out pelvis movements similar to those of women during dancing. When there is dancing at an Indian wedding, men too swing their hips. Their hip movements are similar to the belly dance. Italian men dance Pizzica or Tarantella, which roughly means "dancing life." Syrthaki is the name of the male dance of Greece, and in Turkey and Egypt men dance the Baladi or Beledi, a type of belly dance.

The movements of belly dance are beneficial for men in the same ways that they are for women. It is likely that the Sumerians already knew that a loose and flexible pelvis is good for male potency. Besides physical causes, relationship conflicts and psychosomatic aspects play a decisive role in erection problems and impotence among men.

Many men who suffer from erectile dysfunctions feel stressed and under pressure. Men who endure constant stress in their work tend to tense the pelvis and breathe shallowly, leading to a lessened circulation in the pelvis. Add to that the fear of not performing during sex, and often men will experience erection difficulties.

The male erection is a reaction of the parasympathetic nervous system. The parasympathetic and the sympathetic form two nerve networks that work together to create an erection. If there is a problem with one or both of these nerve groups, men will have erectile problems.

The parasympathetic system slows down body processes: the heartbeat becomes calmer, breathing deepens, and the internal organs—especially the pelvis—receive more blood. The more relaxed a man is, the more active the parasympathetic nervous system will be, making it easier to get an erection.

On the other hand, constant stress and fear influence the sympathetic nervous system, the nerve network that increases bodily processes. Breathing quickens, the heartbeat increases, and external muscles receive more circulation. The sympathetic system mobilizes the body for fight or flight; if those energies are not released, there is overstimulation, leading the body to become tense. This can result in high blood pressure and excess adrenaline. When the sympathetic nervous system is overstimulated, it is difficult for a man to get an erection.

Just as with women, shimmies can help men to loosen tense muscles and relax the body. By teaching how to breathe into the pelvis, belly dance supports the parasympathetic nervous system and teaches bodily relaxation. Some urologists have had good success with strengthening the pelvic floor to solve erectile dysfunctions. Shimmies and pelvic waves are especially good at strengthening the pelvic floor. The strengthening of the pelvic floor can also help to prevent bladder and prostate problems.

certain illnesses were cured in the temples with female secretions. It was considered a special honor for a man to marry a woman who had served as a priestess in the temple for several years. As initiated women, these priestesses understood the deepest energies that drive human existence. Having spent their time in the temple using their bodies as well as their minds to worship the Great Goddess, priestesses understood how to bring together the spirit and the body for a more holistic existence. They understood that spirituality does not exist on a separate plane from corporeality. Rather, the body and spirit exist together in service of the goddess.

The festival of the holy wedding, the *hieros gamos,* during which men and women came together in sexual union, symbolized the wedding of the goddess Ishtar with her son, brother, and lover Tammuz. Furthermore, this sacred marriage was echoed in the temple practices of Aphrodite, where priestesses and worshipping men celebrated love and sensuality through sexual union. This idea of sacred marriage, preserved from the worship of the ancient goddess, appears even today in popular discourse. These celebrations were meant to teach men and women not to use their sexual desires to exert power over the other sex. The woman and man should both give their sexuality and reproductive powers to a higher whole, to the Great Goddess and creation. In other

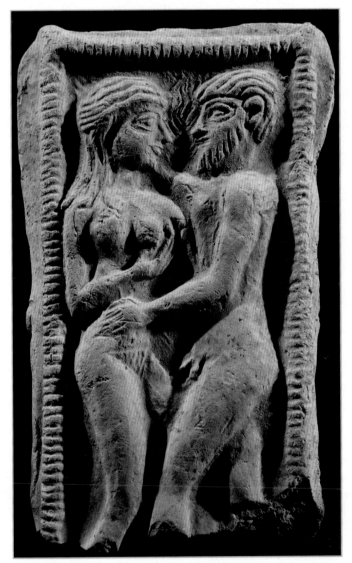

A couple embracing in hieros gamos. Terracotta votive bed, 2nd millenium B.C.E., Susa, Iran. Photo courtesy of Erich Lessing/Art Resource, NY.

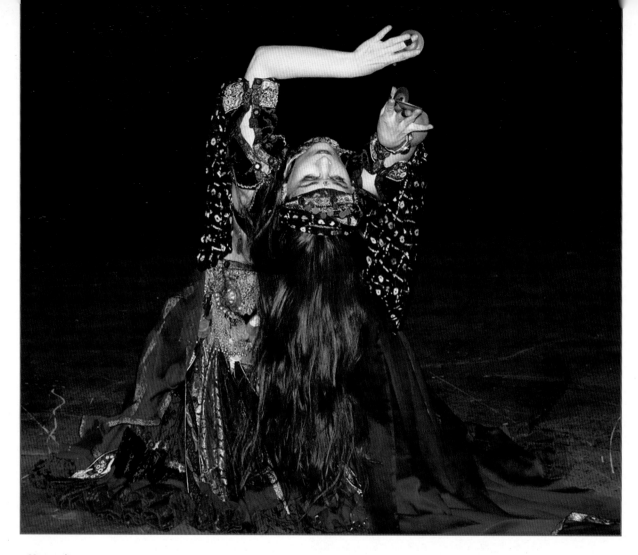

words, connecting to the goddess meant finding wholeness in partnership and creating new life and energy through union.

The belief in the fulfilling power of sexual energy exists in Hindu and Buddhist sexual tantras as well, in which it is suggested that the energy experience during sexual union has the power to propel both partners to spiritual ecstasy. The female partner possesses wild, life-giving shakti energy, which the man needs to fulfill his goal of enlightenment. To discover this energy within themselves, women must be connected to their bodies and the powers that reside therein. The celebration of the holy wedding, like the rituals of sexual tantra, brought the sexes together and allowed them a sexual encounter free of shame and guilt. Men and women were considered equals. The celebration was about the uniting of the two poles, the male and the female, to a whole.

In examining these ancient myths, we see both how dance became an important way of expressing devotion to the gods and goddesses and also how the goddess, woman, and fertility were considered to be connected. These stories are important to preserve and remember because they tell of the power of the sacred feminine, the life energy that controls the cycle of the harvests, fertility, and death. By tapping into this energy to perform the ancient belly dance, women can connect to this great creative/destructive power and release the sacred feminine energy within. They can ground themselves within their bodies and truly feel divine life energy coursing through their veins. Belly dance offers the dancer increased awareness of her physical body and the spiritual implications of the energy that runs throughout her core.

Belly Dance as the Dance of Birth

It is likely that the ancient high cultures such as the Sumerians and the Egyptians had more knowledge about medicine than has been passed down in writing. In particular, it is thought (and has been proven) that belly dancing helps in the birth process. Considering that the dance has strong connections to fertility rites and the Great Mother Goddess, its practical application in the birth process is not that surprising.

From time immemorial, humans have sought to make childbirth as safe and comfortable as possible. A woman who dances is well in touch with her body. Furthermore, she develops her abdominal and pelvic muscles, which aid in a more comfortable and safer delivery. The movements loosen the body so that the woman can relax and open herself not only during

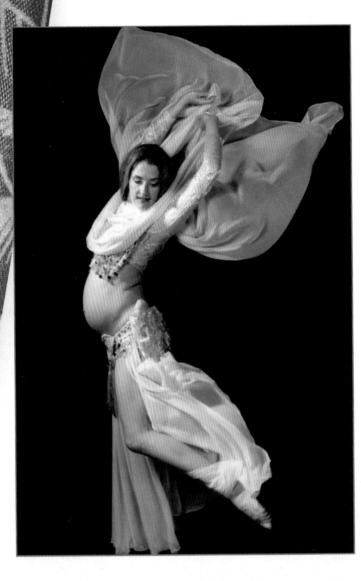

Lynette dancing close to term. Photograph by Julie Faisst.

sexual encounters but also during childbirth. The early cultures thus used dance not only to allow women to celebrate their sexuality and perhaps increase their enjoyment of the sexual encounter but also to make childbirth easier and safer. Among the Berbers in the remote regions of the Atlas mountains, the belly dance is used as the birth dance to the present.

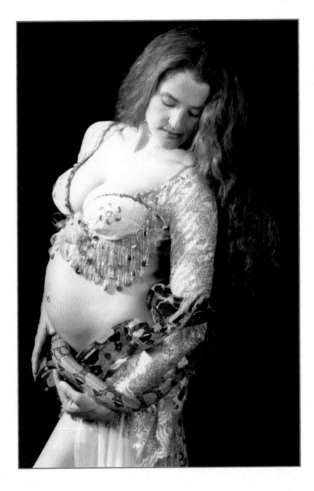

Lynette dancing with boas Bacchus and Meshugina. Photograph by Julie Faisst.

Leading belly dancer and ethnographer Morocco recorded her experience watching dance used as a birth practice among Berbers in 1967. Posing as a deaf and mute maid of one of her friend's wives, Morocco entered the birthing tent for the beginning of the ritual. The women of the tribe spent the day in the tent, eating, drinking, dancing, and singing. The pregnant woman danced for at least half a day. In the center of the tent, in the ground, a small hollow had been made. The next morning, when the birth began, Morocco arrived to see the pregnant woman squatting over the hollow in the ground. The rest of the women formed three circles around the pregnant woman, moving together in a clockwise motion while slowly undulating their abdomens, in a movement that Morocco describes as being "much slower than a flutter." Every few minutes the pregnant woman would stand up and perform the abdominal movements herself. According to Morocco, the woman was very calm.

At noon, the entire dance stopped for prayers and tea. Less than half an hour after the noon lunch break, the pregnant woman squatted in the hollow and delivered her twins, fifteen minutes apart. During the birth, the woman's abdomen undulated in the same way as the dancing women's abdomens moved around her. The dance directly imitated the birthing movement needed for a quick and easy delivery.

There are many elements in pregnancy gymnastics that resemble aspects of belly dance. As we can see in the birth observed by Morocco, the movements of the dance mimic the movements used in birth. Dancing can help pregnant women prepare for birth by becoming more comfortable in their bodies and using their abdominal and pelvic muscles.

For women, the physical insecurities of puberty are often reawakened during pregnancy. Many women don't think they can handle a pregnancy or fear miscarrying. Many loathe their growing breasts and bellies, afraid they are losing control over their bodies and their lives. They worry that their bodies might be harmed by the baby or that they won't be able to lose the weight they are gaining. Advertising images put further pressure on women, causing them to see motherhood as a test rather than as an exciting new experience. Many women feel alone or misunderstood by their husbands. These experiences increase self-doubts and the fear of loss.

By putting a woman more in touch with her body, belly dancing allows a woman to confront her fears and reconnect with the naturalness of the birth process. Practicing the movement she might use during labor and strengthening the appropriate muscles can help a woman feel stronger and more sure about the upcoming challenge. With this preparation, women can reclaim the sacredness of the birth process.

Of course, not all movements of belly dance are appropriate during pregnancy. Shimmies, for example, have limited suitability, since excessive vibration could lead to bleeding in the early stages of pregnancy among women who do not usually exercise. But a woman who already knows belly dance has a good understanding of her body and can judge which movements are good for her and what her limits are.

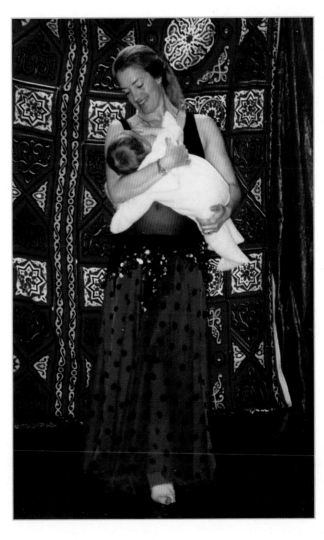

Baby Sophia and Lynette take a break from rehearsing. Photograph by Najia Marlyz.

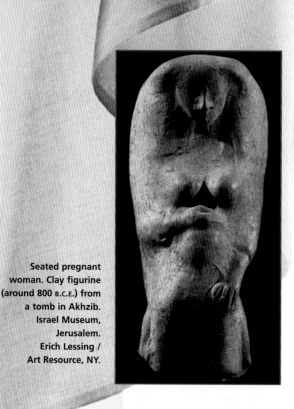

Seated pregnant woman. Clay figurine (around 800 B.C.E.) from a tomb in Akhzib. Israel Museum, Jerusalem. Erich Lessing / Art Resource, NY.

It can be a beautiful experience for a pregnant woman to dance in a group with other pregnant women under the guidance of an experienced teacher. The natural energies of pregnancy, the spirit of giving life and the trust in life come back to the surface. The thought of performance becomes irrelevant as the joy in celebrating new life takes center stage. The unity of the group helps overcome feelings of isolation, especially in cases where a family or partner offer little strength for a woman.

A woman who is able to enjoy her pregnant body is inspired to nourish her body in an appropriate way. And every woman who wants to become pregnant can use the belly dance to gain confidence in her femininity.

During birth there is often a moment when the woman begins to panic. The resulting pelvic and abdominal tension can lead to long contractions, pain, and increased sensitivity. During this type of acute stress, a woman can make herself tight, holding her breath or only taking shallow breaths up to the point of hyperventilating. Practicing belly dance during birth can help a woman calm herself and undo the effects of such panic moments. The slow circulation of the pelvis is well suited for taking deep breaths and concentrating on opening the cervix and moving the baby out of the womb. The key factor is letting go and working with natural contractions. The woman who Morocco observed giving birth mimicked natural movements to most successfully move her twins from her womb.

Each birth has its own pace and its own dynamic. Rather than getting concerned about how long a birth is taking, a woman can delve deeply into

BELLY DANCE: CONNECTING TO THE EARTH

the birthing process, moving her body to natural rhythms. In belly dance, the movement called the stomach flutter can teach women how to breathe while moving the muscles of the pelvis in ways necessary for birthing the baby. This exercise is good for avoiding panic moments, especially when contractions are coming in quick succession or the cervix isn't dilated enough to allow the woman to begin pushing, the dilation being necessary to make sure the baby has a safe passage through the birth canal. In these situations a woman can use belly dancing movements to relax the pelvic region and open herself more fully to allow the baby out of the womb.

In the last phase of birth, a good feeling for the pelvis and strong pelvic muscles are especially important. A woman can "ride" birth contractions more intensively when she has a strong inner feeling for working with the muscles of her pelvis. These muscles push the baby deep into the pelvis and into the birth canal. In this manner, a baby can often be born within two or three intensively supported contractions.

We have found that the belly dance made the births of our children beautiful and harmonious events. Seeing birth as a holy, natural process that the female body is made to perform rather than as a stressful challenge can help women to enjoy and appreciate the sacred moment. Preparing the body through belly dance allows women to connect to their wombs and to work with their bodies during the birth process.

Harems and the Belly Dance

As far as can be discerned, belly dance has traditionally had a special place in the female-only harems of the Middle East. Women learned the dance not only to please their husbands and masters but also to amuse themselves and, as already discussed, to aid in the birth process. Harem life attracted much Western fascination, in part because entry to the harem was forbidden to outsiders. The harem was the subject from which

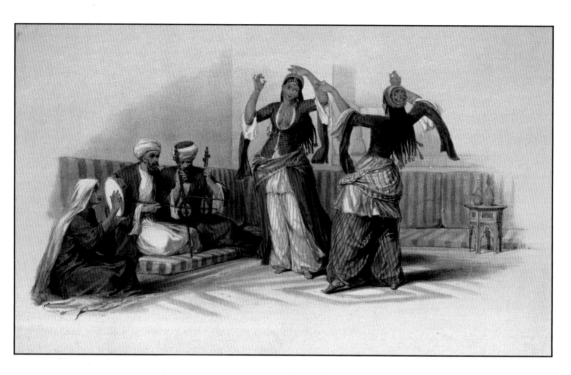

The Ghawazee, or dancing girls of Cairo. Lithograph by David Roberts, 1838/39. From David Roberts and William Brockedon, Egypt and Nuptia, London (F. G. Moon), 1846–49.

Orientalism, fantasies of the Orient that serve the hegemonic west, took root and grew.

There are few "insider" portrayals of harem life; one of the most interesting and revealing is the work of Princess Djavidan Hanum, a European woman who married the last khedive of Egypt.

The khedive was dethroned by the Europeans in 1914. The ruler, who had been educated in Europe, was enlightened and modern. In private, he and his wife interacted as equals and had a happy marriage, but for the outside world they had to keep the appearance of a traditional marriage intact. Djavidan Hanum lived apart from her husband in a harem, where she resided separately with her staff. Although Djavidan Hanum did not belong to any religion, she became a Muslim with marriage. In her special situation she began to deal intensively with the position of women in Islam, especially in the ruling houses.

Hürrem, Companion to Süleyman the Magnificent

Süleyman the Magnificent ruled the Ottoman Empire from 1426 to 1466. During his reign, the sultan strengthened the empire into a world power, centralizing a large and diverse state. As a part of his centralization scheme, Süleyman expanded the *devisirme* system, in which boys and girls from the Christian provinces were taken to Istanbul and raised in the court. The boys became soldiers and government officials. The girls lived in the harem and many married the soldiers and government officials. These government officials were completely devoted to the sultan and the Ottoman state because they lacked any other family loyalties.

Süleyman married Hürrem (or Roxelane), a girl originally from the Christian Balkan states. Most Ottoman sultans never married, so his choice to marry Hürrem, as well as his surviving love poems to her, demonstrates Süleyman's affection for his wife. Hürrem and Süleyman had several children together, including a son, Selim. However, Süleyman had an older son, Mustafa, from a different woman in his harem, who stood to inherit the throne. Needing her son Selim to become sultan so that she could achieve the power and prestige that came with the title of Queen Mother, Hürrem schemed with the grand vizier Rustem Pasha to accuse Mustafa of planning a rebellion against the sultan. Convinced of his son's guilt, Süleyman had him strangled, making Hürrem's son Selim his heir. In 1466, Selim ascended the throne; unfortunately, his mother had died several years before, leaving Süleyman with a broken heart.

In the harem of the Topkapi Palace in Istanbul, there lived over five hundred women. In a harem of this size, many events were hidden from the sultan or could not be explained by him. Power relations changed frequently and the sultan often had to take into account the wishes of the powerful women of the harem. The story of Hürrem illustrates the power available to women in the harem despite their inaccessibility to the outside world.

BELLY DANCE: CONNECTING TO THE EARTH

In her book *Harem*, published in 1930, Djavidan Hanum vividly illustrates how the original teachings of Mohammed were distorted over the course of history through interests driven by power and politics. Originally, love and respect for women played an important role for Mohammed, much as is the case in early Christianity. Love was considered the foundation of a marital union. During Mohammed's lifetime, women had the same right to a divorce as men. Reasons for divorce for either party were incurable illness, alcoholism, impotence, infertility, denial of God, infidelity, refusal to engage in intercourse, or if one party no longer loved the other. If a man tried to force a woman to keep up a marriage even though she no longer loved him, Mohammed himself would enact a divorce. If the man were no longer able to provide for his family, this too would be considered grounds for a divorce.

A woman alone had the right over her body, and even female slaves had the right to refuse themselves. In Djavidan Hanum's words: "All these clearly explained and constant fundaments of Islamic beliefs were corrupted over time by scrupulous sheiks and spiritual leaders according to the wills of the men who paid their salaries, and it was they who turned the original teachings of Mohammed into a wrong and unjust religion. There is no longer a line back to the original teachings out of this mix of what is allowed, disallowed, a sin, this labyrinth of superstition, practices and norms" (from *Harem*, p. 18).

In her book, Djavidan Hanum argues that women lost their rights as Islam was reinterpreted by male clerics and lay leaders. Djavidan Hanum sees the development of the segregated harem as emblematic of the problems with Islam. Belly dance, originally a fertility ritual and a birthing tool, was also affected by the idea of the harem. Within the harem and societies supporting the idea of sex segregation, belly dancing may have become sexualized. Outside of the harem and outside of the Near and Middle East, fantasies of the harem definitely sexualized belly dancing, creating fantasies of an extremely sexual dance done only by women to win favor with powerful men. While women still danced for their own

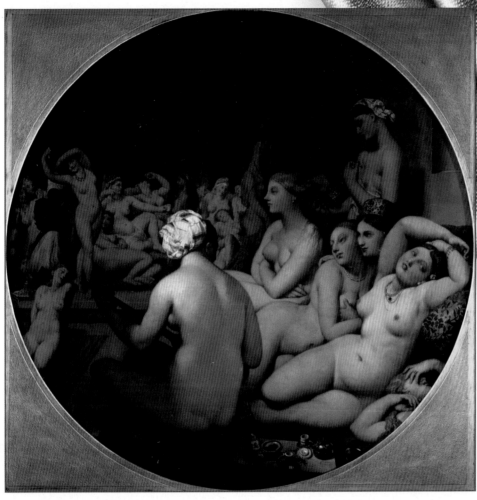

The modern image of the harem has been strongly influenced by the art and writings of the nineteenth century. *The Turkish Bath*, Jean-Auguste-Dominique Ingres, 1862. Paris, Musée du Louvre.

enjoyment, we can see the initial move toward the eroticization of the dance. In attaching a sensual, surface meaning to belly dance, men attempted to strip the dance of its spiritual meanings and power. Like the story of Salome, the scenario presented by Djavidan Hanum suggests a recasting of female spirituality as base and corrupted when compared to male-dominated religions.

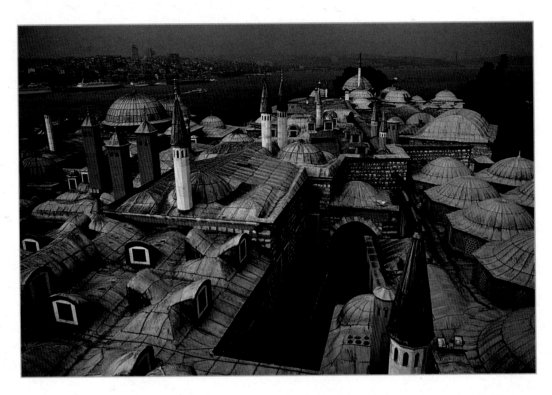

The harem of Topkapi, Istanbul.

The Turkish word *harem* comes from the Arabic *haram* or *haruma,* meaning "off-limits," "disallowed," and "illegal," but also "holy" and "unbreakable." The Kaaba in Mecca and the entire area surrounding it was considered a harem, a safe area. The harem, like asylum in a temple, granted protection against extradition, imprisonment, or death. In this sense, *harem* once stood for freedom. But rulers used harems for the exact opposite purposes and misused the term to identify a place in which women could be sequestered for an unlimited amount of time, hidden from the outside world. In the Western mind, the harem became a complete fantasy land. Because Western observers could not visit the harem, it became the source of many rumors and fantasies about the East and Islam. Most of these fantasies involved scantily dressed women waiting around to sexually please the sultan. Belly dancing, still performed by women within the harem to entertain each other

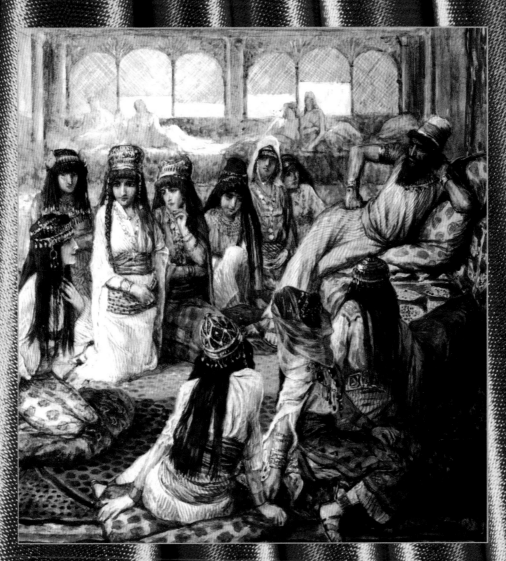

James J. Tissot,
*Solomon and His
Harem*, ca. 1896–1902.
Gouache on paper,
The Jewish Museum,
New York.

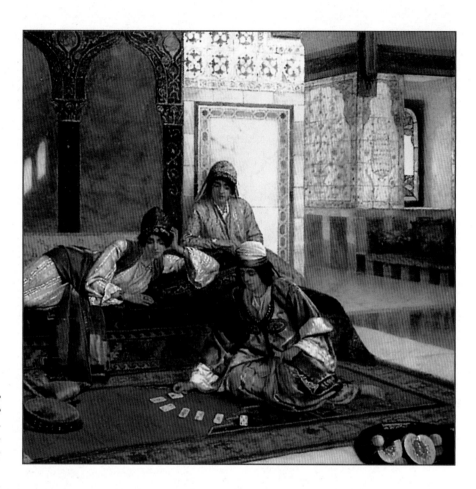

and celebrate special occasions, became known only as a dance of seduction. In fact, most women would never consider dancing in a mixed-sex environment, except perhaps at a wedding.

The size of a harem showed the wealth of the ruler. The first four caliphs, the so-called raschidun ("those who walk the right path") were still legitimately elected—in contrast to those who were to follow. As guardians of religion they received no money for their position. They prayed, fasted, and lived off alms. But the caliph Muawijah later

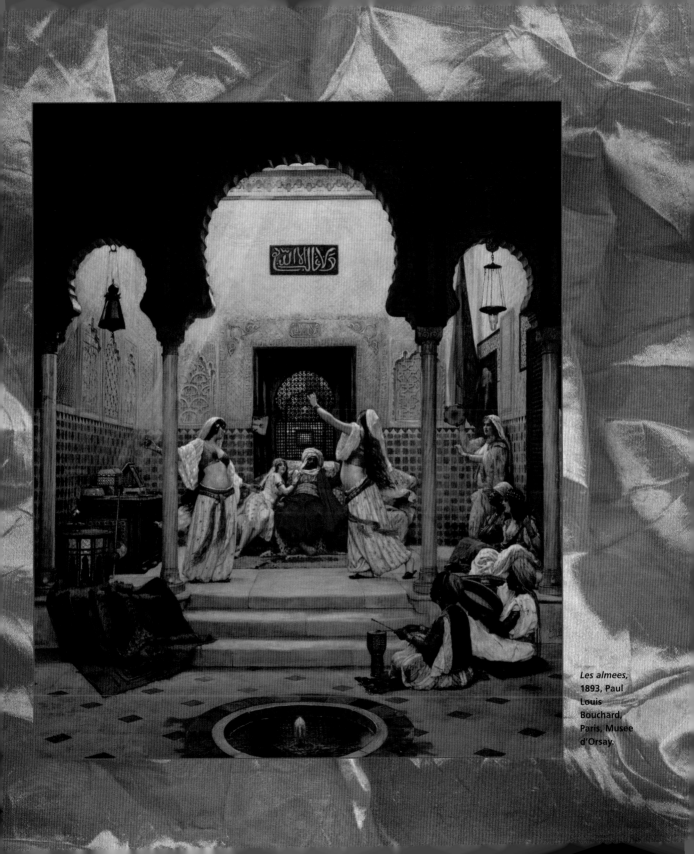

Les almees,
1893, Paul
Louis
Bouchard,
Paris, Musée
d'Orsay.

illegitimately crowned himself the fifth caliph and first sultan and made the position of caliph hereditary. He had his residence in Damascus and founded the first *serial* (another word for harem, or a female-only living space). He introduced salaries for spiritual leaders and thus laid the foundation for the abuse of power and corruption.

The woman that had the most power in the harem, usually the queen mother, had the most difficult and dangerous job of the state. Leading a harem required more skill than being the closest advisor to the sultan. Women that had found favor with the sultan were called *chasseki,* the "most favored." To reach this position the woman had to give birth to a son for the sultan. Since the fate of these women was dependent on the fate of the sultan and they stood to lose their security and comfort should the sultan fall, women interfered in governance, spied, and spun intrigues, doing everything they could to secure their positions.

Prejudices against Belly Dancing

At the 1893 World's Fair in Chicago, a dancer named Little Egypt performed a belly dance with a group of women. The performance caused a public scandal, with the press describing "terrible movements." One of the origin stories about the term "belly dance" is that the term came from the headline "When Bellies Dance."

In many ways, the prejudices against belly dancing in the West date from 1893 and the Chicago World's Fair. At the fair, "the Algerian Dancers of Morocco" performed, the most famous of whom became "Little Egypt," also known as "Fatima." The woman's real name was Farida Mazar Spyropoulos. For the first time, Middle Eastern women came to America and performed (the "Algerian Dancers" were indeed from Algeria), and Westerners could build on extant Orientalist assumptions in watching these authentic dances. The exhibit "A Street in Cairo," which featured camels, bazaars, and dancers,

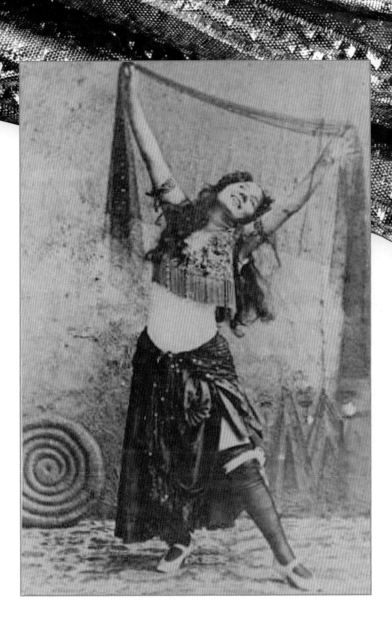

A cabinet card of the famous Little Egypt. The card was put out by Newsboy of New York, and is a risqué shot for the times.

made the most money at the fair. Indeed, this exhibit in a large part helped prevent the fair from losing money. However, many society ladies complained about the dancing and attempted to close "A Street in Cairo."

The exposure of belly dancing to a Western audience led to the continued popularity of Orientalist myths. Wearing scanty, inauthentic costumes,

Understanding the Myth

Our intent in exploring the various origin myths of belly dance has not been to conclusively point to a historical moment from which we can trace the dance. Instead, we have tried to present a survey of the stories and inspirations behind the dance as well as a history of how it has been depicted in both the Islamic and Western worlds.

In her article "In Search of the Origins of Dance," Andrea Deagon makes the important point that more than anything else, origin stories explain what the dance meant at a particular historical moment. Sumerians, Mesopotamians, Greeks, and other peoples have used the dance to venerate the creative/destructive Mother Goddess. Early biblical authors and scholars may have used the dance to denigrate goddess-worshipping traditions through the character of Salome. Orientalists used the dance to project fantasies on to the Middle East and therefore create a political and social hierarchy and proclaim the superiority of the West. Berbers and other peoples have used the dance for birthing.

Today, dancers have a large group of myths and stories from which they can draw their inspiration. In surveying and explaining these myths, our hope is that a woman will find a myth with which she identifies and will elaborate on her identity through her dance practice.

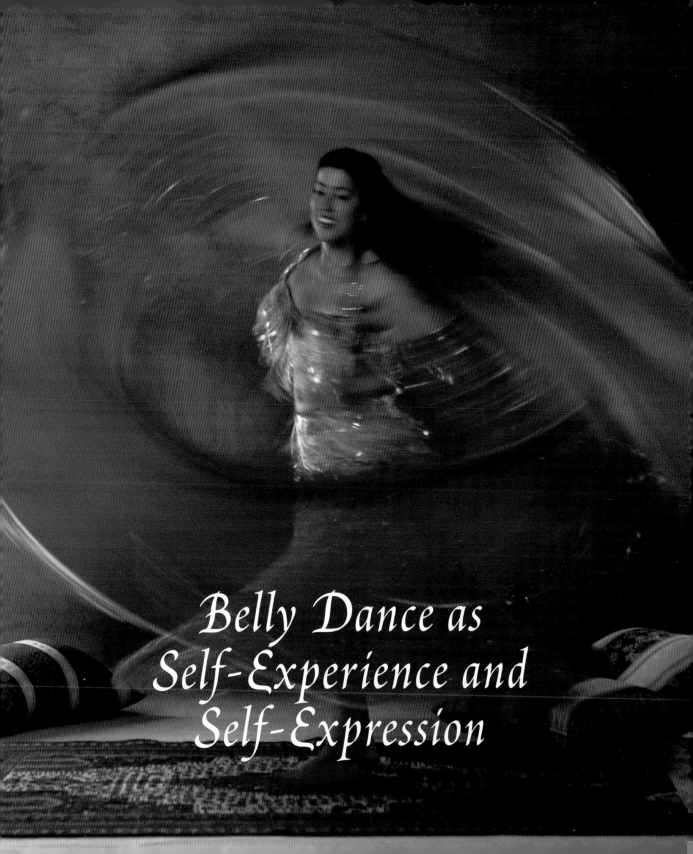

Belly Dance as
Self-Experience and
Self-Expression

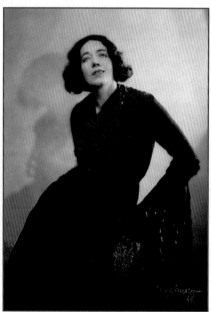

As we discovered in examining the myths that can inspire modern belly dancers, by moving the body dance helps to free the soul. Visionary dancers such as Mary Wigman, Isadora Duncan, and Rudolf van Laban looked to Eastern traditions when crafting new expressions of dance during the nineteenth and twentieth centuries. In Germany, Fe Reichelt, master student of Mary Wigman, contributed to this development. "Laban [a system of movement analysis] views dance in the sense of a complete immersion into the 'flow of movement,' a medium that penetrates all of our activities. . . . At dance and play, practical aspects take a back seat. Play calls up mental energies, and in dance the spirit gives direction."

Dance can help a woman develop a physical relationship with herself, bringing an important element into the circle of self that we call wholeness. Movement improvisation brings to the surface and gives expression to hidden parts of the soul. It has a beneficial effect on personality because it allows a person to more clearly recognize, and thus integrate, various aspects of the self.

In this part of the book we will more closely explore the physical and emotional benefits of belly dancing. Belly dance strengthens muscles and the cardiovascular system, but it also releases energy and encourages its free movement throughout the body. Belly dancing aids women suffering

Visionary dancer Mary Wigman (1886–1973).

from menstrual problems and can help ease the transitions from one life stage to the next. In exploring the spiritual and physical benefits of belly dancing we can see how the dance heals the dancer and how, by dancing, a woman can connect to her innermost life energies.

The Interactions between Body and Soul

Physical and psychological processes influence one another—that is the starting point of psychosomatics. Feelings such as fear or happiness cause certain physical reactions. For example, happiness causes the heartbeat to quicken and the body to feel light while fear causes breathing to become irregular. A fearful person lifts her shoulders, tenses her pelvis, presses her lips shut. Pain begets difficult emotions and changes moods. Certain movements can release memories long stored in the body's tissues. And through our posture we can change our moods: a proud posture creates a proud mood.

The body has its own memory: in muscles and in tissue, a lifetime of experiences is stored. Mental positions and beliefs are lived in the body. The posture of someone who is depressed is different from the posture of a happy person. Constant mental pressures eventually leave physical traces; over time, these pressures can lead to permanent changes on the biological level, and physical symptoms—such as chronic headaches or asthma—may follow.

Both genetic predispositions and events in a person's life can cause illnesses. Stress plays a key role in illness. Aside from excessive exhaustions in job and daily life, other stress factors occur in particular life situations. These situations cause strong emotions and thus require us to adapt. Examples of these situations include births, weddings, separations, divorces, moving, changing jobs, and the death of a loved one. Heightened sensitivity and lack of resources make it more difficult to process these events in a meaningful way, and psychosomatic illnesses are often the result.

BELLY DANCE AS SELF-EXPERIENCE AND SELF-EXPRESSION

Of course, a flexible and sensual body is also a very important source of strength. Belly dance in a gentle but comprehensive way strengthens the whole body and harmonizes the psyche through its positive influence on a woman's feeling of self-worth.

UNDERSTANDING THE MESSAGES OF THE BODY

Intervertebral disc problems and sciatic problems can often have psychosomatic causes. In our search for praise and recognition, oftentimes too much pressure is put on the shoulders. The job of the intervertebral discs is to allow for mobility and flexibility. When we are too tense, our discs can become compressed, causing excessive back pain and tightness. On a mental level, this could mean that there is a lack of openness and flexibility in our lives. Many idioms of speech reflect the relationship between internal and external posture: a person can be labeled "straightforward and upright" or "spineless." The spine allows for an upright posture; it is what gives strength and mobility. Movement practices such as Pilates and yoga seek to strengthen our cores and lengthen our spines and thereby relieve some of this pressure.

Joints give the body its mobility. To become too set on something in our lives oftentimes goes hand in hand with stiff joints, a symptom signaling that the joints have lost their functionality. A stiff neck often accompanies mental stubbornness. Those who tear a tendon or dislocate a joint possibly have a tendency to overextend themselves in other ways as well.

Psychosomatic symptoms occur when we are not balanced in other parts of our lives. Belly dance increases the sensitivity of the dancer to the subtleties of her body's messages. She learns to respect her body and to look after it. In the same way that psychological therapy has effects on physical symptoms through its influence on the mind, belly dance influences the mental state of being via the body.

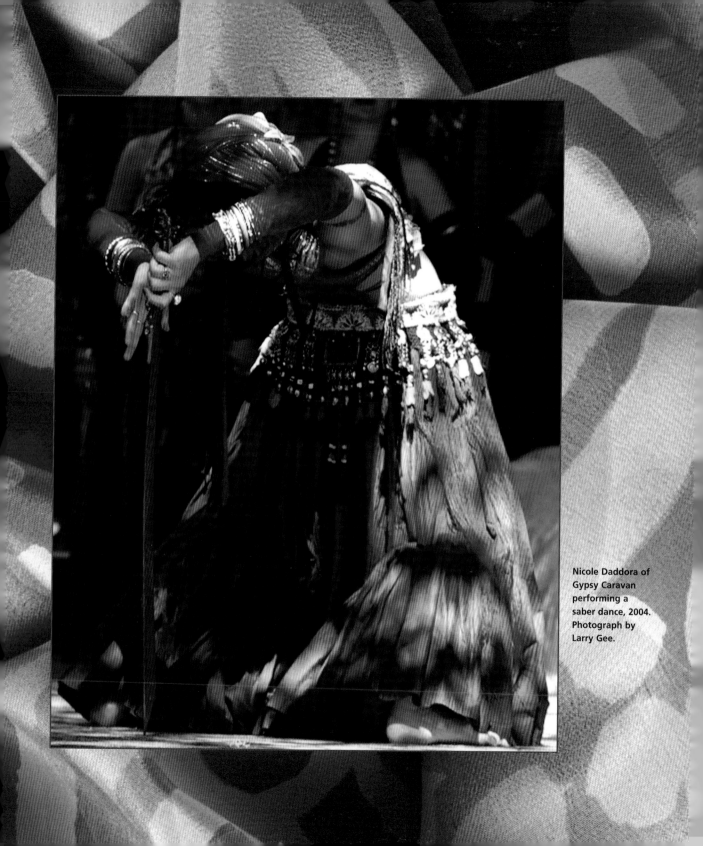

Nicole Daddora of Gypsy Caravan performing a saber dance, 2004. Photograph by Larry Gee.

ILLNESS AS A SIGN OF IMBALANCE

In the fifth century B.C.E., Hippocrates argued that body, soul, and spirit must be brought into the best possible harmony. For Hippocrates, health was the result of a double balance: the internal balance of the body's humors and the external balance of the body in relationship with the environment and the cosmos. Any disturbance destroys the harmony and leads to illness.

Health and illness are relative terms; there is no such thing as complete harmony or complete health. Thus, illness can't simply be considered an "ill": it is always also a sign of an imbalance and the attempt to recreate this

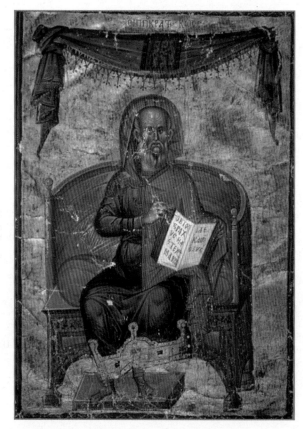

Hippocrates holding his manuscript. 14th century. Snark/ Art Resource, NY.

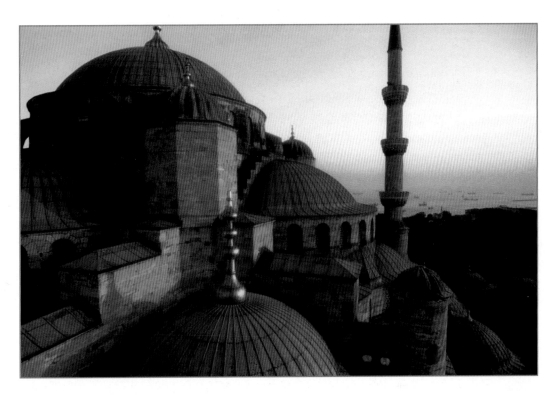

balance by showing us that something isn't right. It is up to oneself to understand this sign and make the necessary adjustments.

In the West, illness was viewed as God's punishment for a life of sin, with recovery being dependent on the strength of one's belief in God. In contrast, in the East meditation and physical exercises played an important role in the healing of physical illnesses. The Middle Eastern philosopher, doctor, mathematician, and poet Ibn Sina (980–1037 C.E.)—also known as Avicenna—wrote the *Canon of Medicine* (Al Quanum fi al-Tibb). This work was well known across the Orient for centuries. Ibn Sina recommends a holistic view of healing: "We have to keep in mind that one of the best and most effective treatments is to strengthen the mental and spiritual powers of the patient, to encourage him to fight, to make his environment friendly and pleasant, to allow him to listen to good music, to bring him together

At a time when doctors in Europe enjoined priests and monks to cure illnesses through prayers, touch, and exorcisms, there was a high level of medical and scientific knowledge in the Middle East.

with people he loves. . . ." Ibn Sina argues that for a patient to heal, his emotional and physical needs must be tended to. Dance, in particular a grounded dance such as belly dancing, provides this complete healing. As the body gradually strengthens, emotional strength is also gained because the dancer becomes sure of herself and her body's abilities. Moving energy around her body makes her feel light and free.

Hara: The Source of Strength below the Navel

The center of the body as well as balance of the body play an important role in physical therapy and Eastern medicine alike. A woman "living in her center" is considered a person in mental balance. In Eastern philosophy, the hara, which is located about two centimeters below the navel, is viewed as *the* source of strength. In Indian philosophy this point is called the root chakra, the place where sexual energy is stored in the body. As other chakras (energy points) along the spine are opened, this vital life energy can move throughout the body, rejuvenating and healing the body and spirit. Health comes only when this chakra is unblocked and energy can move.

Blocked chakras cause both physical and emotional problems. In Buddhist body theory, the entire body is viewed as a collection of channels through which subtle energies of the body move. The most important channel, the central channel, runs directly along the spine. At death, a practiced meditator can disperse through the fontanel of the skull the powerful energies that course through the chakras, thus consciously leaving the body and positioning the self for a better rebirth. Manipulating this energy leads to a breaking of barriers and an opening of the mind. As the subtle channels open the body becomes more fluid and light, freeing the person from harmful accumulated and clogged energy and opening the energy pathways for unencumbered engagement with life. Exercising the pelvic

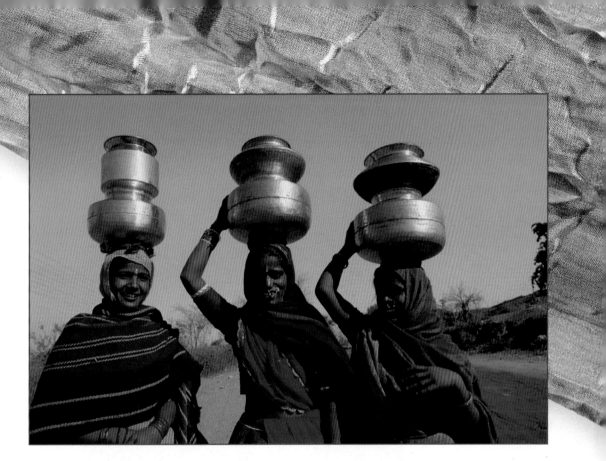

In rural regions of Africa, South America, and India, women to this day carry vessels on their heads. This practice encourages walking from the pelvis—the flexibility of the hips helps the body keep its balance.

area with belly dance movements allows for the vital area at the base of the spine to open, freeing the flow of energy in this important area.

In Eastern martial arts, the goal is to focus on the center of the body and develop movements from the hara. The pelvic movements of belly dance support the hara, having a beneficial effect on mental balance according to Eastern medicine. Belly dance helps us find the center of the body.

The basic positions of tai chi, another hara-based movement practice, are identical to those of belly dance. When she dances, the belly dancer allows energy to flow from this vital life center, enhancing and enriching her health and energy levels.

This vital life energy is often represented as a snake that uncurls and moves up the spine, which is why it is not surprising that some belly

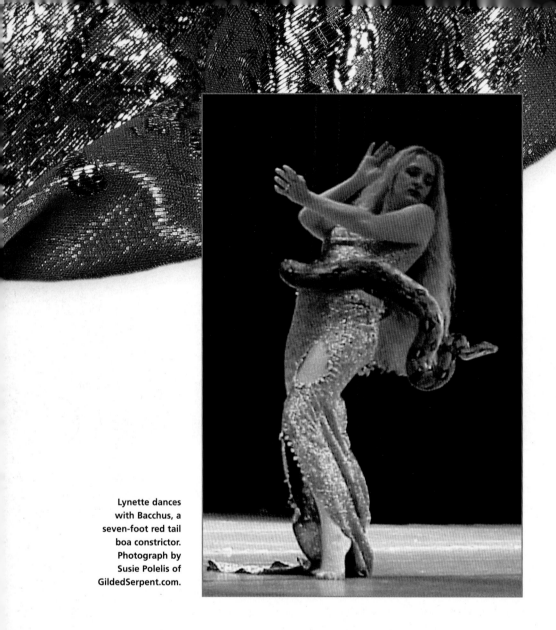

Lynette dances with Bacchus, a seven-foot red tail boa constrictor. Photograph by Susie Polelis of GildedSerpent.com.

dancers choose to work with snakes. Their fluid movements inspire the dancers to open the root chakra and allow their energies to flow. In ancient India, Egypt, and Greece, snakes were connected to the gods and goddesses and were therefore seen as divine. In India, the *nagas,* snake kings of the earth, guard treasure in underwater palaces and keep the books of mystic knowledge. In Egypt, the snake symbolized the goddess. In Greece, priestesses consulted snakes for spiritual and political wisdom. Snakes symbolize the internal sexual energy represented by the goddess, and some dancers choose to dance with a snake to demonstrate the significance of the sexual energy to the flowing belly dance. Kundalini energy, sacred sexual life energy, is often represented pictorially by a coiled snake. This is the energy that you will feel flowing through your chakras as you gracefully dance.

Snakes, moving in a flowing manner, can show a dancer how to open herself and allow her natural energy to flow up her spine. The snake represents the Great Goddess and is therefore a living tie to the ancient goddess cultures from which belly dance originates. Dancing with a snake allows some belly dancers to loosen their bodies more effectively and know the goddess more completely. Remember, however, that a snake is a living creature and therefore must be treated with respect and dignity. Choosing to dance with a snake is a hefty responsibility, one that must be researched and completely understood. For those dancers who do choose to work with snakes, dancing with a snake brings absolute understanding of the power of the goddess and the movement of kundalini energy.

Belly Dance and the Natural Rhythms in a Woman's Life

Despite the women's rights movement and the positive developments in childbirth practice—with midwives again playing an important role in the birth and fathers becoming more involved in the process—women often still lack confidence about their bodies and are easily made insecure or accept a passive role when facing pregnancy. In the Dark Ages the practices of midwives were viewed as inimical to Catholic beliefs, and their work was viewed with great distrust. Clerics feared that midwives might educate women about their sexuality. During the witch hunts of the Middle Ages,

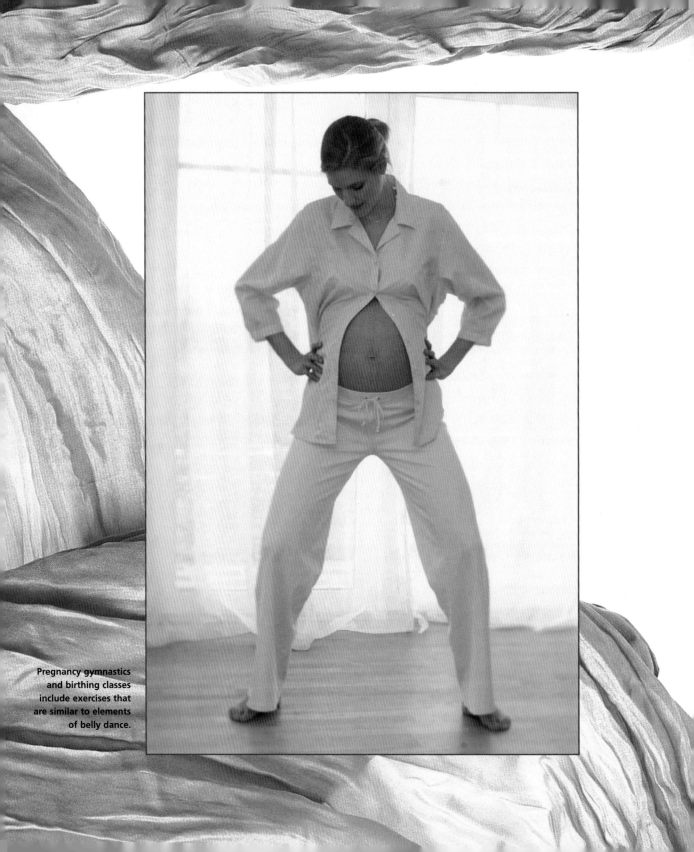

Pregnancy gymnastics and birthing classes include exercises that are similar to elements of belly dance.

midwives were especially vulnerable because of the ancient knowledge of pregnancy, birthing, and the female body that they possessed.

Up to the beginning of the twentieth century, many doctors refused to treat fever among infants, as fever was considered to be God's punishment for a woman's life of sin. Toward the end of the nineteenth century, the United States Congress, at the request of the American Medical Association, banned midwives from assisting in childbirth. In excluding women from the birth process, male doctors began to dictate norms in support of medical intervention rather than allowing the body to perform a natural function. Women became separated from the birth process, facing anesthesia and surgery performed by male doctors.

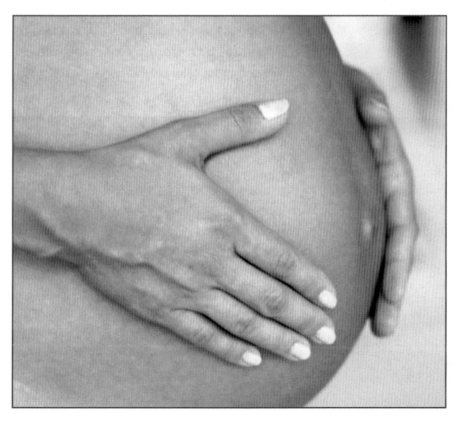

Pregnancy—joy from growing life.

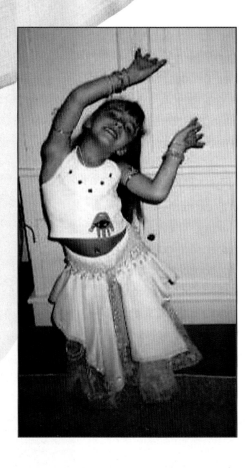

Malak, a young dancer from North Carolina, at her first performance, playing her new zills and wearing the costume her mom made for her.

sense of self-worth. They reject their bodies out of a feeling of not being loved enough. It is in this phase of life that many teenagers develop eating disorders such as anorexia and bulimia. This mental uncertainty and the feeling of being abandoned can also lead to women trying to regain control over their feelings through controlling their bodies. Too many girls fall victim to psychosomatic illnesses in this way. They lack support from their families but they also lack alternative solutions for their problems.

For a woman who is acutely anorexic or bulimic, the movements of the dance might be too much and might pose a health risk. But if a woman has worked through her illness in therapy, belly dance offers a good way to regain contact with her body and to rediscover and accept her femininity without judgment.

THE MENSTRUAL CYCLE AS A RHYTHM OF NATURE

Many women tend to see the monthly moon cycle—the menstrual period—as negative, something akin to a necessary evil. This often leads to neglecting one's own cycle. But through the monthly bleeding the body cleanses itself and prepares for the next cycle. Women who can't accept this aspect of their femininity often suffer under the physical changes that precede the onset of their period.

Women who are under a lot of pressure at work tend to contract their pelvises. This can make menstruation very painful. Here, too, it is good to heed the messages of one's body; when a woman has disorders related to her monthly cycle, she should consider the disorder as a symptom of imbalance in her life and attempt to correct it.

Amenorrhea, the absence of a period, can signify the rejection of one's role as a woman. It also occurs when a woman loses too much weight and so commonly occurs in anorexia. Dysmenorrhea, painful monthly bleedings that might be accompanied by migraine, cramps, nausea, or metabolic problems, could signify anger toward the body and the female within. Premenstrual syndrome (PMS) is often a reflection of a rejection of female life processes. The main physical syndromes of PMS are pressing and pulling pains in the lower abdomen several days before the onset of the period; tension from the belly to the legs and breasts; headaches; water retention around the eyes, feet, and hands; flatulence; and constipation. Psychological symptoms are nervousness, irritability, emotional fragility, aggression, depressive moods, feelings of fear, and troubles sleeping, as well as chronic exhaustion.

BELLY DANCE AS SELF-EXPERIENCE AND SELF-EXPRESSION

In the case of endometriosis, which is caused by parts of the mucous membrane of the uterus sloughing off, traveling into the intestine, and causing colitis during the monthly bleedings, disappointment and frustration is expressed on a physical level. The lack of self-love is often replaced by an excessive consumption of sweets.

Many women unconsciously carry over societal norms or the behaviors of their mothers. They see menstruation as something dirty and try to suppress it. Dealing with old myths and the cultural roots of the belly dance helps remind modern women that menstruation was originally seen as something positive and was very respected. After all, all of life has a cyclical rhythm: that is the essence of the story of Ishtar and Tammuz. When women accept this law of life they can accept their own cycles. They can allow themselves peace, protection, and withdrawal before the onset of their periods without seeing their needs as a sign of weakness. Then they can enjoy menstruation, the moment in which tension in the uterus is released.

Many women feel sexually excited during their periods but do not dare act on their feelings in fear of rejection. In the cultures that honored the Great Mother, there were initiation rituals for girls when they had their first menstruation. The girls connected their menstruation with happiness, joy, music, and dance. But today, many mothers that want to convey to their daughters a positive attitude feel alone and don't know what to do. Belly dance connects women to their cycles and opens the pelvic regions. Mothers looking to express a positive feeling about menstruation might try dancing with their daughters to signify the important and valuable life change that puberty represents.

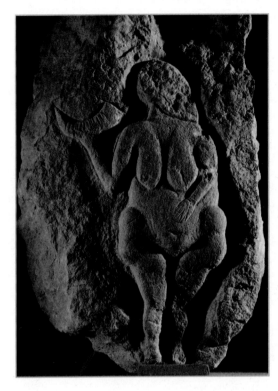

The famous Doni of Laussel, a 26,000-year-old limestone relief found near Marquay, Dordogne, France. Erick Lessing/Art Resource, NY.

SEXUALITY: OPENING ONESELF DURING THE ENCOUNTER

An important feeling for women who suffer from sexual problems is helplessness and fear that they must place themselves at the mercy of the man. One of the most common sexual dysfunctions among women is the so-called appetence dysfunction—that is, a lack of sexual desire. Many women have a hard time seeing their lust as something positive. They are afraid of being misunderstood or having moral judgment passed on them. This attitude makes it more difficult to open up and offer themselves during sexual encounters. The only positive aspect that they see from their sexual encounter is that men desire them and therefore they have some small

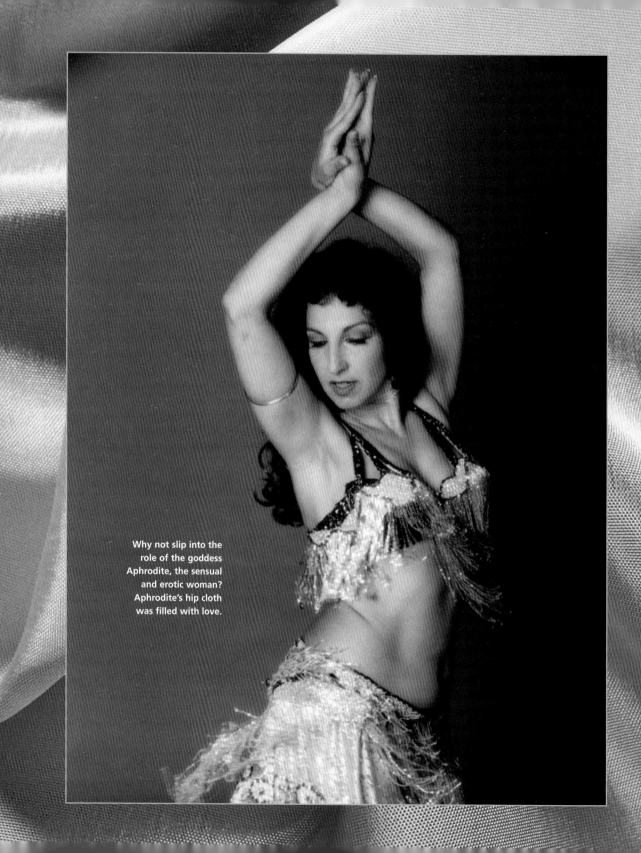

Why not slip into the role of the goddess Aphrodite, the sensual and erotic woman? Aphrodite's hip cloth was filled with love.

amount of power over the man. However, these women soon discover that the ability to orgasm is linked to opening oneself in the encounter and letting go of egoistical feelings, something they cannot do if they are focused solely on the power dynamic of the relationship.

In the orgasmic experience, the line between man and woman is dissolved, and the two become one for that moment. This transformative moment is recognized in Hindu and Buddhist tantras and also in the hieros gamos ritual discussed earlier. In becoming one in bliss, both partners can

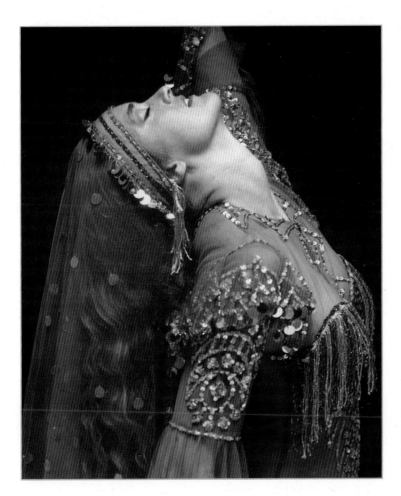

Lynette in balady (beledi) dress. Photograph by Bob Giles.

open their bodies and allow healing life energies to flow between them. It will be hard for someone who does not feel respected as an equal by the opposite gender to trust in someone and shed their fear of being hurt. Without dealing with these fears, a woman cannot open herself to the transformative power of the sexual encounter.

In the case of sexual problems, traumatic events from childhood and youth—events such as sexual abuse, physical abuse, or rape—can play a role. Many women who have such a history have a difficult time accepting their bodies as beautiful and healthy, even after psychotherapy. Despite these problems, they feel the desire to be with a man. In belly dance, women can heal their bodies. They experience their chest and pelvic areas completely independent of a sexual context. Through these dance movements a woman can build new confidence in her body and give it proper attention. It is not her body that is at fault for these painful experiences—rather it is the fault of those who did not respect this soul and this body.

The protected environment of a belly dance circle can be very healing. It is a healing experience to move in an erotic and seductive manner for joy and fun, without having to worry about pleasing a sexual partner. Many women are afraid of being the subject of moral judgments if they move in erotic ways. A woman who is passive during sexual encounters will experience sexuality in a more painful way and may tense up because her pelvis is not moving in rhythm with the movements of the man. But a woman who knows the strength of her legs, her pelvis, and her vagina does not have to fear male sexuality.

BELLY DANCE AS AN IDEAL COMPANION FOR MENOPAUSE

Many women begin belly dancing during menopause. At the midpoint of life, their summary of lived lust and sensuality is not always positive. Now is the time to make up what you missed and to give your body more attention. Many physical and psychological ailments of women during

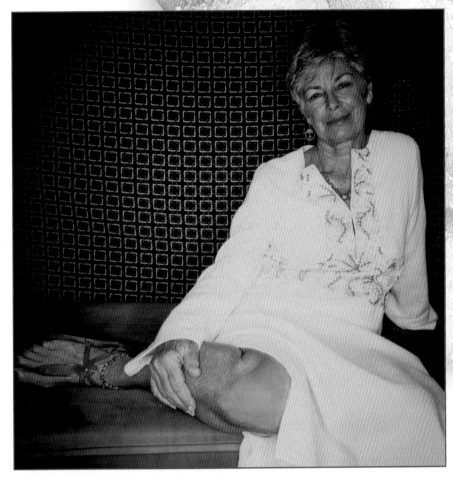

The movements of belly dance are ideal for the mature female body. All the organs affected by the hormonal changes of menopause are strengthened by increased blood circulation.

menopause can be positively influenced by belly dancing. In our narcissistic world, where the youthful and smooth body is considered beautiful, there are few affirmations for the mature body.

When the children have grown and left home, many homemakers start getting the feeling that they are now really living life on the sidelines and are no longer needed. But it is exactly this time in life that might be the chance for a new orientation, for example to take time for your own body again or to discover new hobbies. If a relationship ends at the same time, there is the danger that the woman will give up altogether, questioning herself and all that she has done. This thinking amplifies fears and depressive moods. Of course there are big hormonal changes going on within a woman at this time, but by nature she has become used to working through these changes and to adapt to new situations. If the mature woman trusted her body, she would know: the experienced female body has a special erotic quality.

The Sensual, Creative, and Erotic Aspects of Belly Dancing

In belly dancing a number of basic figures can be combined in many different ways. A woman can give in entirely to the dance and to her feelings. There are no set step sequences, since at its core the belly dance is essentially a dance of improvisation. Especially in Egypt, famous dancers created artistic choreographies. Yet it was their personalities that gave each choreography an individual face.

Westerners are especially inflexible in the pelvis. Many people's stature reflects the military ideal of good posture: stomach in, chest out. This posture was reinforced by the antisexual Puritanism from Victorian England. Thus we have to work hard to relearn the natural and easy flow of walking from the pelvis, which the people of some cultures do so naturally. In rural regions of Africa, South America, and India, women carry loads on their heads, as when they are carrying water pots to or from the well. This encourages walking from the pelvis and increases flexibility at the hips.

We in America and Europe do not know this means of transporting goods—at least not anymore. Belly dance is a good way of rediscovering the pelvis and its flexibility. It helps us find a feeling for the balance of our bodies. Standing with legs slightly spread and with knees slightly bent

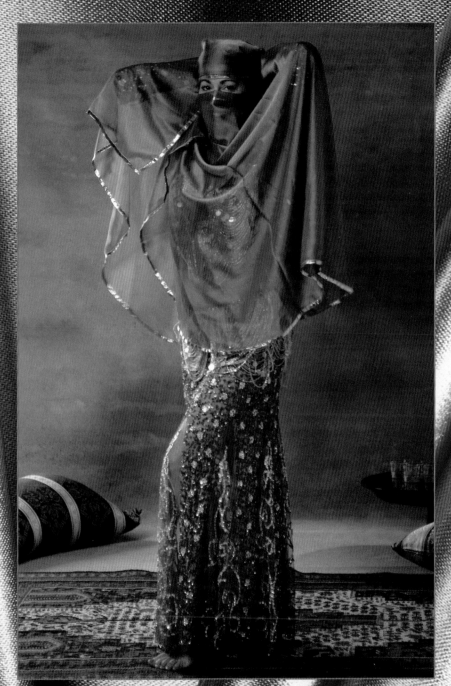

The sensual pose of a belly dancer.

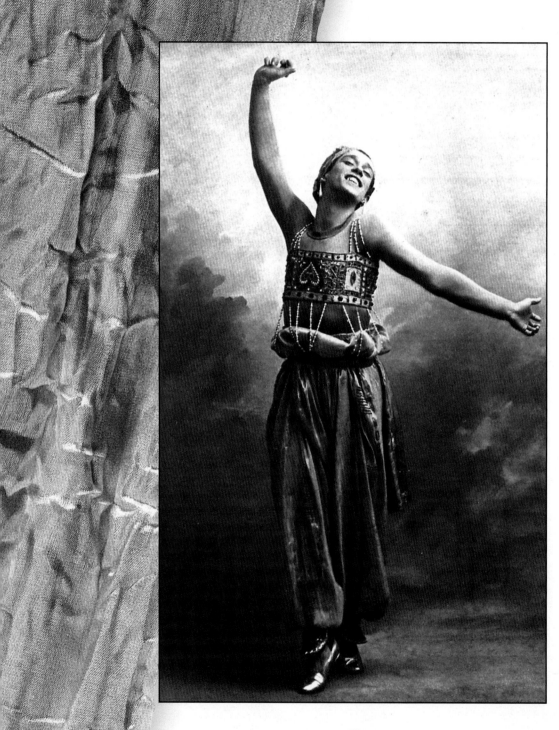

Vaslav Nijinsky as the Golden Slave in "Schéhérazade," ca. 1911.

BELLY DANCE AS SELF-EXPERIENCE AND SELF-EXPRESSION

allows for a more steady stance. When the pelvis is loose, breath can travel through and deep inside the body, ensuring an optimal supply of oxygen for our internal organs. Finally, this well-grounded stance does not compress the spinal cord but instead maintains its optimal flexibility.

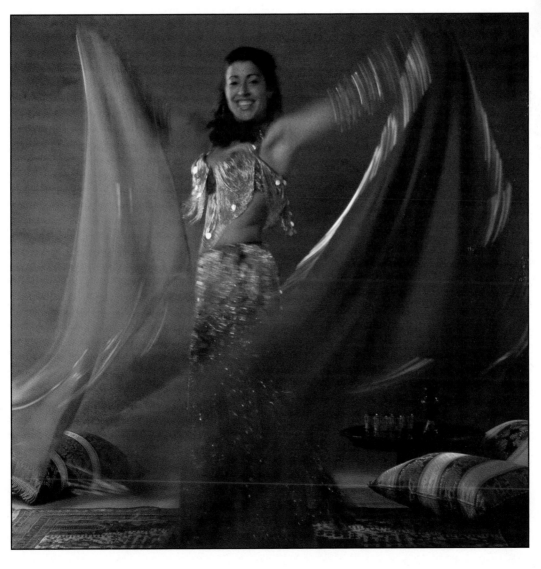

BELLY DANCE AS SELF-EXPERIENCE AND SELF-EXPRESSION

Before you move on to the specific belly dance movements, take a moment to consider the physical, emotional, and perhaps even spiritual imbalances in your own life. How might your dance practice empower you? In your reflection, consider the role of your story, the myth that you would like to express through your dance. You could borrow from the origin stories discussed earlier or you could create your own myth, the myth of your own life. Belly dance allows you the freedom to move and create, opening your body to powerful energy flows and healing your imbalances. Remember to let yourself explore the possibilities as we move into the practical aspects of the dance.

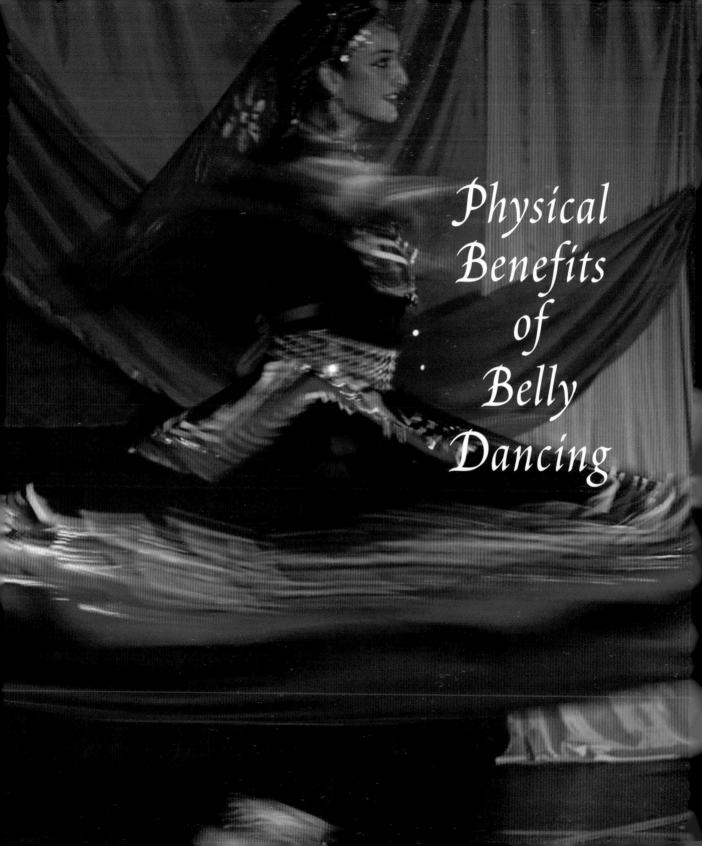

Physical
Benefits
of
Belly
Dancing

*A*s with any other cardiovascular exercise, belly dancing can be used to maintain a healthy metabolism and to increase energy. Those who spend the better part of the day standing or sitting often complain about having slow metabolisms. When the metabolism is slow, weight begins to build up and water is easily retained. Belly dance stimulates the metabolism and helps to detoxify the body. By dancing, a woman can work on her physical form while connecting with her inner spirituality.

To achieve a strong and toned body, you should ideally spend forty-five minutes three times a week practicing belly dancing in addition to attending class at least once a week. By working on your dancing with this degree of commitment, your muscles can build up slowly and remain in shape.

Many women have a hard time practicing dance at home because they don't think they can find the time. Overcoming this obstacle demands creativity. Dance with your children for ten minutes at night before putting them to bed. If you have a baby, put the baby on a blanket and dance for her. Infants love music and movement and they enjoy finger games too—all arm movements and steps with a veil can be mesmerizing for a baby. Even a teething, crying baby can often be soothed this way.

You can listen to music and practice hip circles while you cook dinner. If you work at a computer for hours on end, allow yourself a break every now and then to loosen your shoulder and arm muscles with shoulder shimmies and hand circles. Finding ways to bring dance exercises into your everyday life can help you do good things for your body in the middle of your daily routine.

When you allow yourself more time to exercise, you can vary your exercises, improvise, and let your body guide you.

In looking at the essential elements of belly dance, we hope to give a basic understanding of how the body moves in the dance. Dance in front of a mirror to give yourself feedback on your posture and movement sequences. We recommend this to correct mistakes that may creep in from the beginning days of your study; however, if you have the feeling that the mirror is leading you to examine yourself critically and is thus distracting you from dancing, then trust your bodily intuition and dance for yourself.

Throughout history, belly dance has been used to connect with something much deeper than superficial ideas of achievement. Yet discipline, performance, and the drive to succeed are a tripartite foundation at the core of Western culture. Most people in our culture have a hard time letting go of their competitive nature and allowing themselves to experience life without urging forward in an effort to achieve success. In beginning belly dance training, though, it is important that you allow yourself to perform the movements without worrying about doing them "perfectly." Remember, you dance for yourself—to connect with universal energies, to understand yourself, and to heal your body. The ancient dancers were connecting to the inner goddess and derived great power from their knowledge of the goddess. Belly dancing enters you into this timeless wisdom tradition.

Take the exercises and dance moves in this book as an invitation to

Dancing body

In the mirror there the image
Of my body naked.
Curved lines, soft curves
Breathe sensuality.
A woman's body,
Groomed and well-formed . . .
There the arm rises,
All muscles are at play,
Nerves vibrate,
And the body becomes an
    instrument:
A leg that swings,
Measuring the room,
A foot that smiles
    condescendingly,
A hand that can weep,
Arms that, full of holiness,
Touch the room.
Tensed chests, bulbous body,
In whose curve the room
    becomes poetry.
Mysterious transformation!
I bow respectfully to the
Body that has become dance.
        MARY WIGMAN (1886–1973)

Belly Dance as Cardiovascular and Strength-Training Exercise

What health effects does belly dancing have? This was the question that a professor at the athletic academy in Köln, Germany, set out to research using electromyography. Professor Fobröse's research showed activity in the trapezius, the long muscles of the back (the erector spinae), and in the abdominal muscles as well as in the buttocks during belly dancing. Regular belly dancing of about sixty minutes not only strengthens those muscles but also strengthens the heart and increases circulation. Thus belly dance can be considered a cardiovascular exercise, having similar effects as jogging or cycling.

A low-intensity dance session recorded a heart rate of 113 beats per minute, rising to 144 beats per minute when the dance went to high intensity. Training for health or body-toning purposes should only be done at low intensities: a workload of 110 to 115 beats per minute is sufficient, especially for people who haven't exercised before. This rate should be maintained for an extended period of time (about 45 minutes). Those who dance in this way will quicken their metabolism and burn more fat. Combined with a sensible diet, it is possible to improve your body shape following this protocol.

Anyone who has ever tried belly dance knows how many muscles are used in the dance. The athletic scientists saw particularly intensive reactions in the abdomen, back, and buttocks. Muscles in these regions reached almost one-fifth of their maximum contraction capacity. The different exercise routines showed that muscles are activated both independently and as part of entire muscle groups.

These movements showed especially strong muscle reactions in the abdomen:

- Hip kick
- Twist

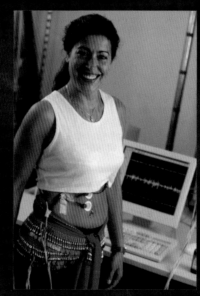

Studying the health effects
of belly dancing at the
athletic academy in Köln.

PHYSICAL BENEFITS OF BELLY DANCING

- Hip circles
- Hip roll

These movements showed strong reactions in the long muscles of the back:

- Hip kick
- Hip circles
- Standing-lying figure 8s

The movement most effective for the main buttocks muscles was:

- Shimmies

The pilot study also showed these other effects of belly dance:

- Belly dancing strengthened the heart muscle and stimulated circulation;
- Belly dancing increased metabolism, especially at low intensities;
- Muscle activities are particularly effective for stomach, back, and hip muscles; and
- High-intensity dancing is appropriate only for experts and well-trained athletes.

Professor Fobröse also examined the reactions of the so-called shawl muscle of the back, the trapezius: this muscle is active in almost all of the above-mentioned exercises, albeit at a very low level.

For a better understanding of how belly dance affects muscles, it is necessary to gather data from a wider sample. However, Professor Fobröse's work illustrates how belly dance can benefit a woman as part of a regular fitness regime, allowing a woman to strengthen her physical body while connecting with her spiritual core.

explore and discover your body. Try to adopt a positive attitude toward your body. If you accept your body and release that acceptance in your movements, the dance will put you in touch with your joy and vitality.

The mental readiness to accept the present moment is a practice common to many meditation systems. The way is the goal. Belly dance is not about being able to complete an exercise perfectly and as quickly as possible; instead it is about feeling the movements and merging the physical and the emotional. Familiarize yourself with your body and with its limits. Give your body time to build up the muscles that you need for the dance. Even if you don't think you're making any progress, your body is learning.

PHYSICAL BENEFITS OF BELLY DANCING

The Basic Stance:
Grounded, Relaxed, Full of Breath

The stance is an important part of the starting posture for belly dancing. The legs should be hip-width apart with the feet parallel and pointed forward. See the box "Exercises for Good Ground Contact" on page 88 for enlivening the feet and to get a good feeling of your connection with the ground.

To develop a relaxed and fluid posture, make a conscious effort to loosen your knees whenever you can. For example, when you are standing in line at the store or waiting for the bus, bend your knees and allow yourself to stand in this more relaxed pose. Although this will feel unnatural at first, you should become accustomed to it over time. Since standing with

The Basic Starting Position for Belly Dance

At the start of each practice session, check for the correct posture.

- Is my head loose and light on my spine?
- Does my neck feel free and relaxed?
- Are my knees slightly bent?
- Is my pubic bone tilted slightly forward and up?
- Is my pelvis open and wide?
- Are my arms hanging loosely from my shoulder joints? Do my shoulder blades drop slightly toward the floor?
- Is my chest raised slightly forward?
- Is my breath steady and slow?

Begin each dance session with this mental checklist. By training your body in the correct posture at the beginning of your dance practice, you lessen your risk of injury. Soon this posture will become natural.

loose knees is better for the knee joints, some sufferers of chronic knee pain may find relief simply from revising their stance this way.

Most people lock their knee joints when standing, holding their legs perfectly straight; it feels strange to allow the knees to bend and to stand in this more relaxed posture. However, to perform belly dance movements the body must remain relaxed and fluid; locked knees prevent smooth hip motions and hinder moving across the room while dancing.

It is important to have a strong basic stance because it will support your body as you learn more complex moves. Make sure that your head is held high, your neck loose and relaxed. Imagine that a string is running through your spine, holding your head up. Make sure that you have a "flat" back; tilt your pubic bone slightly forward and up to soften the curve at the low back. You can check this by lying on the floor with your knees bent, feet flat on the floor. If you can reach your hand underneath your low back, you are holding tension there. Breathe into the musculature along the spine, relax the belly, and work with the positioning of the pubic bone to relax the back toward the floor and flatten the spine.

Your arms should hang loosely from your shoulders and your shoulder blades should hang toward the floor. Don't hold your shoulder muscles tight, as this will cause pain and jerky movements. If you are having problems relaxing your shoulders, do a few shoulder rolls. As you relax your shoulders, open your chest cavity. Imagine there is a string pulling your breastbone up toward the sky. Opening your chest will allow you to breathe slowly and forcefully, which is essential for cardiovascular health.

Tilting your pelvis forward and up as you stand in basic position will help you to keep your back flat when you are standing. Make sure that your pelvic area is open. This may seem uncomfortably open and sexually suggestive, but it is important to keep the pelvic area open to allow for energy flow from within. Remember, keep your knees bent. You need to be able to move gracefully and locked knees will prevent that. Also, locking the knee joints can harm your knees.

Exercises for Good Ground Contact

Curl and straighten your toes a few times. Try lifting your toes up, keeping them in the air, and then lowering them again.

Play with shifting your weight. Move your weight forward onto the balls of your feet. Take one step forward, then return to center. Now shift your weight backward until you're standing on your heels. Take a few steps on your heels. (A slight sound from the heel is no cause for worry—it's probably the release of fluids that have accumulated there.)

Shift your weight to your left leg. Press the heel of your right foot to the floor and turn your heel right and left. Now roll your right foot along its outside edge and back again. The bone next to your small toe might be sensitive to the touch, so don't put too much pressure on this area. This is where the reflexology zones of the shoulders are located.

Transfer your weight back onto the ball of your right foot and draw small circles with the outside edge of the foot while still pressing the ball of the foot against the ground. There are important reflexology zones on the ball of your foot below the toes. A small sound from this area again is no cause for worry; however, if you experience pain in your foot, stop the exercise immediately. Slightly shake your foot and ankle and circle your foot in the air inwards and outwards a few times.

Shift your weight to your right leg and begin working with the left foot.

This posture may seem overly complex and contrived, but making sure that you start in the correct posture every time you dance will ensure that you have a long dancing career that is free of injuries. You will also dance more smoothly and gracefully because you will not be holding tension in your muscles.

Deep breathing, especially the pause between the inhale and the exhale, is very important for calming the body and centering the self. In this pause, the breathing channels relax and the remaining air flows out of the body. We hardly notice this process on a conscious level. The more used air exits the lung, the more fresh air the lungs can take in during the next inhalation. This happens automatically and effortlessly—the more we exhale, the deeper we inhale.

Conscious breathing during belly dance will allow you to deepen your stretches and move with greater fluidity. Make sure that you are breathing as you dance. As you are finding your relaxed stance, take some time to practice deep breathing and breath awareness.

Strength and Grace: The Pelvic Floor

For many of us, the pelvic floor is a forgotten part of the body. The pelvic floor is made up of three muscle layers. The external muscle layer lies directly under the skin and surrounds body openings. The middle layer runs perpendicular to the external layer; when this layer is contracted, the buttocks are noticeably cinched toward one another. The internal layer of the pelvic floor supports the controlled opening and closing of the bladder and the intestines and supports us in walking upright. Strengthening these muscles allows for more subtle manipulations of the sacred energy located in the genital area.

When we are dancing, a strong pelvic area allows for more powerful and graceful movements.

There are two kinds of exercises for strengthening the pelvic floor: passive exercises and active exercises. During passive movement exercises, only the internal muscles of the pelvic floor are consciously contracted; the rest of your body remains at rest. Thus the muscles of the pelvic floor are strengthened without increasing the heart rate, making these exercises very low-stress on the system. They can usually be performed by even those people who need to be careful with movement because of a heart or

The Changing Menopausal Body

During menopause a woman's body produces less estrogen, which can lead to thinning of the vaginal mucous membrane. As well, the circulation of the mucous membrane decreases, causing the membrane to become more vulnerable to injury and infections, including uncomfortable itching and discharge. The active and passive pelvic exercises strengthen the vagina. The conscious contraction and relaxation of the vaginal muscle stimulates circulation within the mucous membrane, making it more resistant to infections and in other ways compensating for the lack of estrogen.

Training her pelvic floor can help prevent the onset of bladder incontinence at menopause. Bladder problems can also be rooted in emotional or sexual issues. Women who are sexually tense and feel that they always have to please their partners are more likely than their peers to develop bladder infections.

Fearful women and women who have low self-esteem tend to adopt a subordinate role in a relationship or make themselves dependent on their partner, and these women can have sexual problems as well. Although they may find safety in their relationship, they are unable to develop sexually due to the dominant role of the partner; they find it difficult to relax and let go physically. Oftentimes they experience anger at their partner, whom they hold responsible for their lack of freedom.

Pain during urination is an indication that the bladder may be in distress. Bladder problems offer an invitation to begin thinking about what anger or pain you might be holding on to in your sacred energy core. Anger, fear, and regret block the vital energy centers of the body and can cause numerous health problems. Since belly dance helps women to reconnect with sacred, erotic energy and to reinhabit their bodies, dancers can use belly dance to more easily understand what life factors may be causing physical problems and then work with the dance to heal their bodies and prevent future problems.

circulatory condition. The passive pelvic-floor exercises can aid in recovering from a hysterectomy or from most general bladder problems. Strengthening these muscles allows women to control their bladders and can make for more enjoyable sex; post-pregnancy, they can help women to heal from the birth process. When you incorporate these exercises into your daily workout routine, you are engaging in effective and targeted prevention against later bladder weaknesses and incontinence.

You can do the following basic pelvic exercise either standing up or sitting down. First, try to really feel the muscles of your pelvic area, the muscles surrounding your vagina and anus. Take deep and steady breaths. It helps to imagine that you have a strong need to urinate. Pull your vaginal muscles inward and then upward, keeping the tension for a moment before letting the muscles drop as you exhale. With the next breath, again pull your muscles inward and upward, thinking that with each breath you

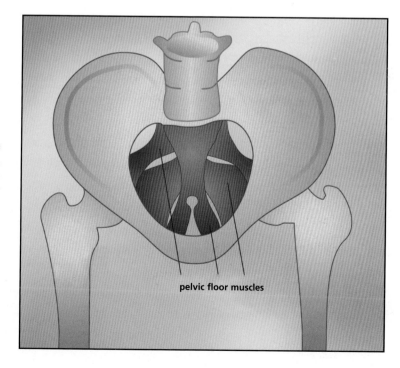

The bones of the pelvis and the pelvic floor muscles.

pelvic floor muscles

are also allowing air to enter through your vagina into your pelvis. Imagine that you can contract your muscles so much that you are closing the external labia of your vagina. Keep this tension, then release. (You can also do this exercise while you are actually urinating, which allows the best chance for getting the feel of the movement—experiment with stopping the urine at various moments.)

You should practice this exercise several times a day to really get in touch with your pelvic floor. Exercise for eight to ten contractions. The passive exercises are great to do whenever you have a few minutes—when you are driving or waiting in line or during your morning commute. By strengthening this area you are controlling one of the main energy centers of the body.

Once you have mastered the basic exercise, you can begin practicing an isolated version, contracting and releasing only the muscles of your anus. First contract the vaginal muscles and then the muscles around the anus. Keep the tension and release. You can contract the anus muscle and the butt cheeks separately from one another. Try to see whether you can clearly tell the difference between the anus and the gluteal muscles of the buttocks.

You can vary this exercise depending on your needs. After some time, you will consciously feel your pelvic floor as strong and alive.

With the active exercises, you are moving your entire pelvic region, exercising the surrounding muscle groups as well. Active movements of the pelvis increase muscle tone and strengthen circulation, thus having a conditioning effect on the body. The wave movements, pelvic circles, and shimmies all fall into this category. These exercises increase flexibility, support rhythmic and coordinated breathing, reinforce the proper positioning of the body's center, and ease menstrual cramps and pregnancy pains. We will go into active exercises in greater depth when we discuss the hips, because hip exercises tend to exercise the pelvic area as well.

Even though we do not exercise or think about the pelvic area in our daily lives, strengthening this vital area will allow for a firm foundation of your

Developing Strong Bones and Bodies through Belly Dance

Osteoporosis, a decrease in bone density that mostly affects women, is a condition that often occurs during menopause. Although the decrease in calcium absorption usually starts years earlier, it is the hormonal changes that accompany menopause that progressively weaken the bones. Loss of bone density increases risks of broken bones from everyday activities.

Osteoporosis can be prevented in a number of ways, such as getting enough calcium and taking a vitamin D supplement. Research suggests that regular exercise and strength training may also help prevent bone loss. It is possible to avoid bone degeneration by training steadily over years. Belly dance as a dance of the whole body is a good and low-stress training for women to prevent osteoporosis. Belly dance is low impact yet provides a solid cardiovascular workout—for example, the vibrating motions of shimmying loosens skeletal muscles and stimulates the circulation of blood within bone tissue. Becoming more familiar with your body allows you to notice changes and hopefully to prevent osteoporosis before it is too late.

dance. Furthermore, strengthening the pelvic area can give you additional health and sexual benefits. Beginning with these small exercises will help you to develop a strong pelvic area and benefit your hips, back, and legs.

Preparing to Dance: Warm-up Exercises

Now that we have considered the basic posture for belly dance, we can move on to exploring our bodies through the dance. As a part of beginning your belly dance practice, we suggest that you attend a class at least once a week with an experienced teacher. Attending a weekly class creates a

Be Careful with Spine or Joint Ailments

While most people can enjoy practicing belly dance movements, it is important to realize your own limitations and construct your dance practice so that it is helpful, not harmful, to your body. The joy of dance comes from your inner movement and your connection with sacred energy. When you move externally in ways that your body cannot handle, you disrupt your energy flow and open yourself to physical injury.

Even if you have no chronic illnesses that limit your dance, you still need to remain conscious of your health when dancing. We all get sick, and these infections need to be taken seriously. The body needs rest until the infection has healed. Increasing circulation to infected joints can contribute to the spread of an infection.

When you are sick, you should carefully consider whether your body needs the healing movement of dance or whether you should instead take some time to rest. Belly dance encourages listening to and understanding the signals of the body, so please don't ignore these signals in the name of practice.

greater incentive to practice in your everyday life. In addition, the company of like-minded women is fun, offers new contact, and can help overcome frustrations with the learning process.

The dance movements that we illustrate and explicate in this book are designed to give a basic foundation in belly dancing. Taking a class with a great teacher can help you build your beginning skills and learn more advanced moves, which are too complex to properly explain in a book. You need to see an advanced dancer move her body gracefully and receive feedback from other dancers to learn the hardest moves.

The one complicated dance move that we have included in this book is shimmying. Even though they are better suited for advanced dancers, shimmies loosen the whole body, even for beginning dancers who are just learning. Don't despair if it takes you a while to learn the shimmies (although some women are able to pick up shimmies surprisingly fast). Shimmies require an exceptionally loose posture, which takes a lot of practice to acquire.

In the next section of the book, "Now We Dance," we will cover dance movements for the entire body and then learn how these individual movements can be brought together into a full dance. The exercises below will help you to prepare your muscle groups for learning the dance.

Do some stretches before the warm-up exercises to make sure your body is warm and your circulation is strong. Shake your whole body, especially the joints. Shake your wrists while keeping your fingers loose. Start slowly and then increase the tempo. Just shake your worries out of your body. Shake your shoulders, your pelvis, your knees, your ankles. During this exercise, breathe in through your nose and out through your mouth. The focus is on breathing out to let tensions or worries flow out of your body. Visualize any negative energies you might be holding flowing out of your skin. You can imagine your dance transforming these energies into a protective white light.

Yawn a few times in a row. Yawning loosens the jaw muscles and increases the circulation to your brain. Be careful with your head! While you are loosening your body, allow your head to nod along slightly, in small movements. Avoid strong or abrupt movements—you might pull something in the tender regions of your spine. While you are loosening your body, keep your mouth slightly open to relax your lower jaw.

Loosen your face. Move your lower jaw left and right with small movements. Consciously and slowly open and close your mouth, like a fish. Try to picture yourself chewing gum: first chew slowly and then more intensively to loosen your lips and the joints of your jaw. After this exercise your face will feel loosened and fresh, and a relaxed face looks more youthful. The jaw, the shoulders, and the pelvis all relate to one another functionally and energetically. When you relax your jaw you are also opening your pelvis

PHYSICAL BENEFITS OF BELLY DANCING

and vice versa. A person who clenches her teeth also compresses her pelvis and has a hard time letting go.

It is essential that you warm up before entering an intense dance practice. Moving methodically over your body will allow you to be sure that all parts of the body are loose and can help you avoid an injury. Try any or all of the explorations below in creating a warm-up for yourself.

STRETCHING YOUR ARMS

Stand with your legs slightly more than shoulder-width apart, your knees loose and relaxed. Your feet should be pointed straight ahead. Alternate raising your arms straight up in the air, raising first your left arm and then your right arm. When you lift your right arm, bend your right knee toward the ground. When you raise the left arm, bend your left knee. Be sure your knee doesn't twist as it bends; make sure the knee stays aligned over your toes.

The stretch of the arm comes from the shoulder. Imagine the stretch continuing all the way into your fingertips. Picture yourself as Tantalus reaching for the grapes that are just beyond your reach. Perform five repetitions on each side.

ROWING WITH THE SHOULDERS

Alternate between pulling up your left and your right shoulders and letting each one drop back down again. Now pull up both shoulders at the same time and let them drop. Let your right shoulder circle forward and then backward; then circle your left shoulder forward and backward. Next, circle both shoulders forward at the same time. Finish by alternately circling the shoulders, as if you were rowing.

Try to perform this movement slowly and gracefully. You can incorporate this movement into a dance sequence, so it should not be jerky and slow. As you move, breathe deeply and imagine energy moving along the spine and into your shoulders. Allow yourself to feel each movement deeply.

HIP CIRCLES

Slightly spread your legs and loosen your knees, keeping your feet parallel and facing forward. Make a big circle in the air with your left hip. Your upper body moves with it to keep you in balance. Imagine you are inside a drum and are stirring thick dough, using your hip as a spoon. Try to enlarge the circles, as though you wanted to touch the edge of the drum with your pelvis.

Circle five to ten times to the left and then five to ten times to the right.

Strengthen Your Back with Bare Feet

Traditionally, belly dance is performed barefoot. Most dancers continue this practice today, which means the floor that you dance on should not be tiled or cold. Also, avoid extremely hard floors that will damage your feet.

Walking barefoot is a wonderful foot reflexology massage and is something that you can do outside your dance practice. It is not only fun but also adds beautiful (and to some women, erotic) sensations to your daily movements. It is good for your body image and can help prevent certain maladies. The feet get air, circulation is increased, and you won't have sweaty feet or ingrown nails because of shoes that are too tight. Walking in high heels or ill-fitting shoes is bad for the spine; walking barefoot every once in a while can be very beneficial for your spine and your feet.

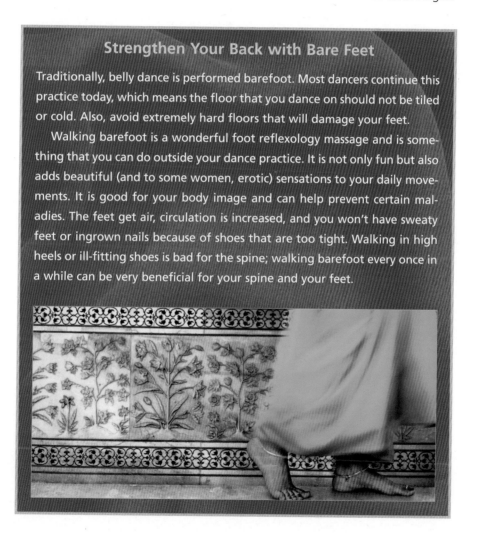

Most dancers notice that circling one way is easier than circling the other way; right-handed people usually find circling to the right easier and vice versa. It is important to practice both directions, however, so that you develop ease of movement and balance on both sides of your body.

ANIMAL MOVEMENTS

Get down on the floor on all fours. The back is parallel to the floor, the hands are shoulder-width apart and parallel to one another, the fingertips are pointing forward. Arch like a cat, tensing your belly and buttocks and lowering your chin to your chest. Inhale and remain in this position for a moment. Return to the starting position as you exhale. Repeat this movement five to eight times.

Next, from the starting position sway your hips back and forth like a duck trying to get water out of its feathers or a dog shaking her tail. Pull in your belly and let it drop again. Keep moving your hips to loosen the muscles. If you want to relax your diaphragm while you do this exercise, try panting like a dog. While panting, your breaths stay shallow and inside the chest.

STRETCHING THE LEGS

For this warm-up, stand with your legs slightly apart, knees bent softly and feet parallel and pointing forward. Bend your upper body forward and stretch your left arm toward your right foot while lifting your right arm behind you. Change sides and move your right arm to your left foot.

Perform this exercise five times for each side. Make sure you feel the stretch in the trunk of your body. Move slowly to allow the muscles to fully extend.

You can also do this exercise sitting on the floor with your legs spread wide. The important thing is the stretch. Take two or three deep breaths to let your muscles relax into the stretch. In the interest of protecting your joints, don't bounce.

GENTLE TRAINING FOR THE ABDOMINAL MUSCLES

Lie on your back with your legs pulled up. Imagining that you're pushing something up over your chest, press your arms up. This movement will slightly lift your upper body off the ground. During the exercise the lower vertebrae remain tightly on the ground.

Repeat this pushing motion eight to ten times. You should feel the stretch in your upper abdominal muscles.

THE HALF-BRIDGE

This warm-up exercise strengthens the thighs and spine. Lie down on your back with your knees bent at right angles and your feet firmly planted on the ground, toes pointing forward. Press your feet to the ground so that your pelvis lifts off the ground; the harder you press your feet into the ground, the more your pelvis rises. Your head and shoulders remain on the ground.

Stay like this for a moment, then roll the pelvis back down to the ground vertebrae by vertebrae. The lower vertebrae are the last ones to touch the ground.

Repeat this exercise three to four times. You should feel this in your lower abdominals. Be sure not to rush the movement and to roll each vertebra down gently. You want to allow your muscles to work; if you move too quickly or bounce, you make the exercise ineffective and you risk injury.

STRETCHING AND RELAXING THE SPINAL CORD

Begin this warm-up in a standing position, legs together and knees slightly bent. Lift both arms straight above your head. Let your upper body fall slowly forward, fingertips toward your toes. Remain in this position for a while to stretch your legs. Don't be frustrated if your hands are far away from the ground—do not bounce your upper body to try to touch the ground. If you incorporate this movement into your daily routine you will quickly notice improvements.

Dressing the Goddess Within

Most women begin to develop their favorite belly dance costumes as they become acquainted with various belly dance movements. Costuming becomes an important part of the dance: veils, belts, skirts, and other clothing can be incorporated into the movements. As you develop a personal mythology and dance practice, feel free to experiment with different types of clothing and styles. Choose costumes that are comfortable, easy to dance in, and honor the goddess within.

For warm-up, sweat pants and a sweater or similarly heavy top are recommended. You need to keep your body warm as your muscles slowly loosen and are preparing for more intense exercise. Once you have properly stretched your muscles and are ready to begin dancing, we recommend yoga pants or a wide skirt with an elastic waist. You want to make sure that your belly is unencumbered. For a top you can knot a T-shirt above the belly; if you prefer to cover your abdomen, wear a body-hugging top. These tops are available at sporting good stores and places that sell yoga clothing. You can also find beautiful belly dance clothing at various online emporiums.

Slowly roll the spine upward, letting your head hang loose until the very end of the movement, when you lift the cervical spine to bring the head to vertical. The more slowly and consciously you straighten your spine, the more your spinal cord receives a chance to rest.

This relaxation exercise can be supported through coordinated breathing. Breathe in as you raise your arms, breathe out as you let your upper body fall toward the ground. Breathe in as you straighten your spine, breathe out as you lift your head.

These next exercises should help to loosen the legs and back and help you become more acquainted with your pelvic area as a life-filled center rather than as a place to be feared.

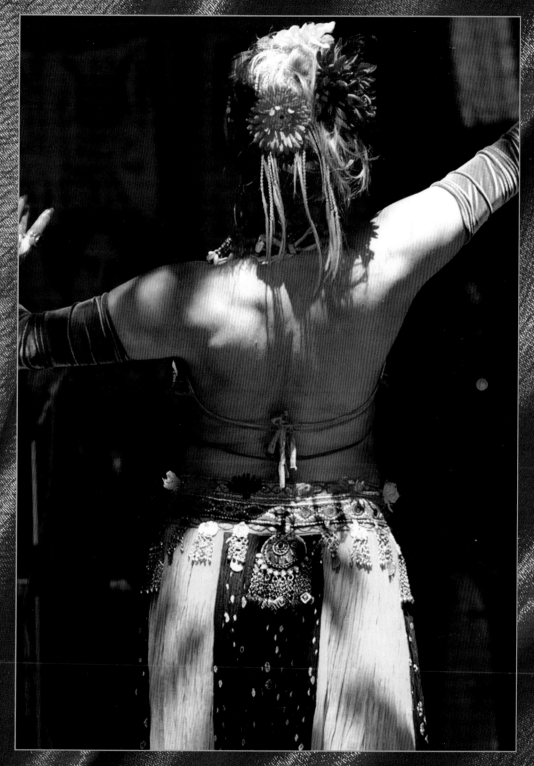

Carol Lindgren
Vance of Gypsy
Caravan performs
at the Oregon
Country Fair, 2004
Photograph by
Larry Gee.

comfortable with the pelvic region as a source of life and vital energies. The movements of the dance draw this energy from its source in the genital area and allow the energy to flow throughout the body. If you are feeling uncomfortable in your dance practice, try this pelvic-circle exercise to see if it will help.

Using a foundation story may help you too. How can the dance help you to become more comfortable within your body? Remember that Artemis, the Greek war goddess, was celibate. Belly dance is less about sensuality and more about recognizing the life energy within yourself. If thinking about sexuality and sensuality makes you uncomfortable, focus on the energy as the energy of life, the energy that allows you to accomplish all the things you do. Becoming familiar with your life energy will allow you to understand how it flows in your body and how you can help it to flow better to live a healthier, more balanced life.

RELAXING THE LUMBAR VERTEBRAE

Use this exercise to conclude your warm-up. You should feel the effects of this exercise in your lower back. It will help you open up the area and loosen your muscles.

Lie on your back with your legs bent toward your chest and your feet and knees parallel to one another. Spread your arms horizontally and then drop your legs toward the right side of your body. Your shoulders and arms stay on the ground, providing a good stretch to the hips. Take a few breaths and then slowly lift and rotate your legs to the left side.

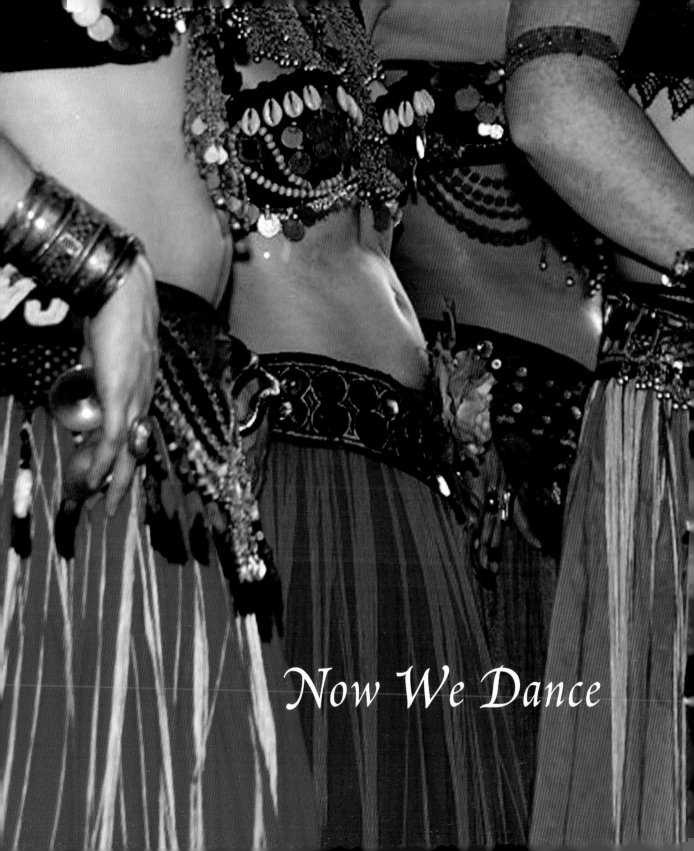

Now We Dance

$\mathcal{I}$n the last section we considered some of the basic information you will need to begin your belly dance practice. The warm-up exercises will help you prepare your muscles and get into a relaxed and peaceful state of mind for your actual dance practice.

Try to maintain the relaxed feeling you achieved during your warm-up. As you dance, maintain flexibility and energy flow throughout your body. Think of your own story to give power and meaning to your movements. You worship the sacred energy within yourself when you dance. Each movement, even if it's not done "perfectly," still honors your sacred energy. Think of the goddesses we discussed earlier: Ishtar, Artemis, and Aphrodite. How might the qualities they embody inform your dance practice? Remember, having an origin myth to think about while you dance can help you to connect the physical movements with the deeper traditions from which they developed. Making this connection can make the dance a more holistic experience for you.

We will now move throughout the body considering the basic dance steps. Some of these movements will be unfamiliar to you and require a lot of practice while others you will likely find relatively easy. If you practice daily, you will progress rapidly in learning the steps.

First Steps

In belly dance, it is important to put proper weight on the feet. The bulk of the weight rests on the edges of the feet. The feet stay flat on the ground. They are spread hip-width apart and parallel to one another. The knees are slightly bent and are also parallel to one another (1). The knees should point neither in nor out as this would strain them. Remember to keep them slightly bent—this keeps the hips loose and flexible. The pelvis is straight, with the spine lifting from the pelvis. The shoulders drop back slightly. Imagine a string tied to your chest that is lifting the chest cavity and spreading it wide. The head is also lifted as if suspended by a string and the chin slightly raised (2). Breathe steadily, the breath flowing deep into your pelvis.

As you allow the breath to flow in and out of your lungs, think of circulating the energy within your body. You are preparing yourself to move energy through your veins and invigorate your spirit. Taking a moment to

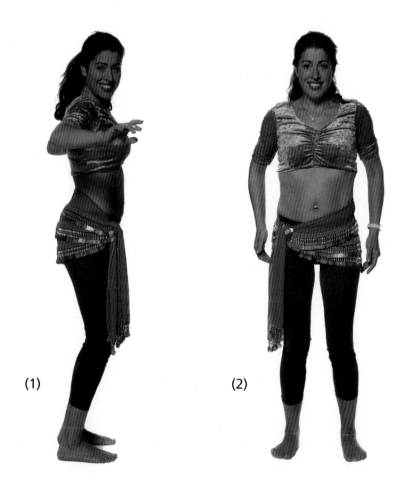

(1)   (2)

properly set your body and take cleansing breaths will allow you to center yourself in the moment and imagine your own story. Belly dance has a long and glorious history of honoring the sacred feminine; you enter into that legacy by beginning your own dance practice. Honor that legacy by preparing yourself to be present in your dance.

Moving the Hips

Starting position for the dance is the basic position detailed on pages 86 and 87. During this movement you can either put your arms on your hips, which will help you feel the movements more intensively, or you can let your arms hang loosely on your sides. You can also hold them as if you were carrying a big, round balloon in front of your body. When circling your hips, pay attention to keeping your knees as steady as possible—your knees should not move with your hips. Many women have trouble at first learning to initiate movements from the hips, which is why we recommend also trying this exercise with a partner: let a friend hold your knees steady so that you can isolate the movements in your hips and thus gain a sense of the range of motion available there.

Remember to think of your hips as a giant spoon that you are using to stir thick dough. Move your hips in a circle, practicing moving in both directions. For the full instructions on this movement exploration see pages 97 and 98.

KICKING THE HIPS

Kick your hip to the left and then to the right as though you were using your hips to push someone aside. This movement should be strong and forceful. Then kick your hip forward (3) and back (4). Some women are embarrassed by this movement as they find it pointedly sexual. But this is merely about loosening your pelvis and is an expression of your vitality. Still,

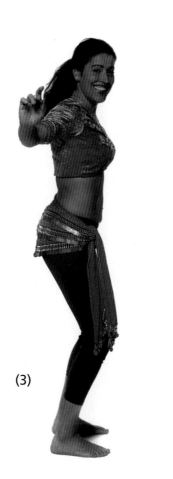
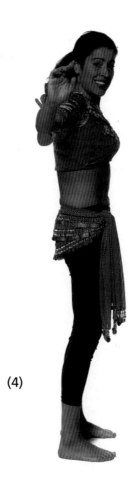

(3)   (4)

if you feel uncomfortable with this movement, leave it out of your beginning practice; you can return to the exercise later. Do this hip kick ten times
in each direction.

SWINGING THE HIPS

The swinging of the hips is the result of intense legwork and weight
shifting.

Shift your weight to your right foot. Lift the right heel and keep your
weight on the ball of your right foot. This movement causes the right hip

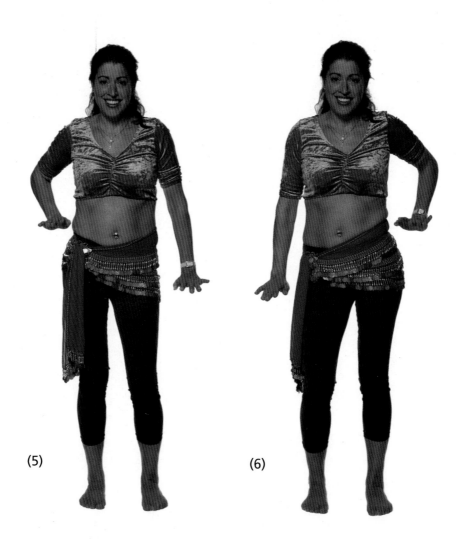

(5)   (6)

to swing upward (5). The left leg lengthens slightly but the knee remains bent; don't straighten your knee to the point of locking it.

Put your right heel back down on the ground. Shift your weight to your left foot, then to the ball of the left foot. When the left heel lifts, the left hip follows (6). The right leg lengthens while the knee remains slightly bent.

Do this movement ten times on each side.

VERTICAL HIP ROTATIONS

During vertical hip rotations the hips move up and down in alternation, like the bowls of a scale. The hip rotation comes from the basic position and is caused only by moving the pelvis. Both feet remain flat on the ground.

Leaving your feet planted and your knees loose, raise one hip and then the other hip. This is a small but intense movement that you should feel in your abdominal obliques, the muscles that wrap around your lower rib cage and waist. You can vary the intensity of your hip rotations by going deeper into your knees or by rising to your toes while rotating. Perform this exercise ten times on each side.

HIP TWISTS

The twist movement is a horizontal hip rotation. During the hip twist the hips move back and forth horizontally while the shoulders and upper body remain steady. Don't forget to breathe. Develop the movement slowly and only increase the speed when you feel comfortable.

To feel the twist, first move your weight to the right leg, then back to the center, and then to your left leg. When the weight is on the right leg, try to see whether you can keep your balance if you lift your left leg and vice versa. Try to keep your knees loose.

Like the vertical hip rotations, this will be a very small but intense movement. Twisting helps you to develop your balance. Perform the exercise ten times on each side.

HIP CIRCLES

During the small hip circle, the hip moves while the upper body remains steady. The thighs support the movements of the hip. Picture yourself standing inside a square; concentrate on touching the corners of the square as you move. Start with small circles and gradually increase the size. Remember to keep your upper body steady.

If that goes well, move from the hip circles inside the square to small pelvis circles. Visualize your pelvis at the center of a spiral; the spiral is tight at the center and gets larger as it circles outward. Beginning at the center, circle the pelvis in a small movement around the spiral, gradually circling outward until the movements are big. The pelvis now moves along the outer edge of the spiral. Then reverse direction and return to the inside of the spiral until the movements of the pelvis are very small again.

Circle right (7) and left (9), ten times in each direction.

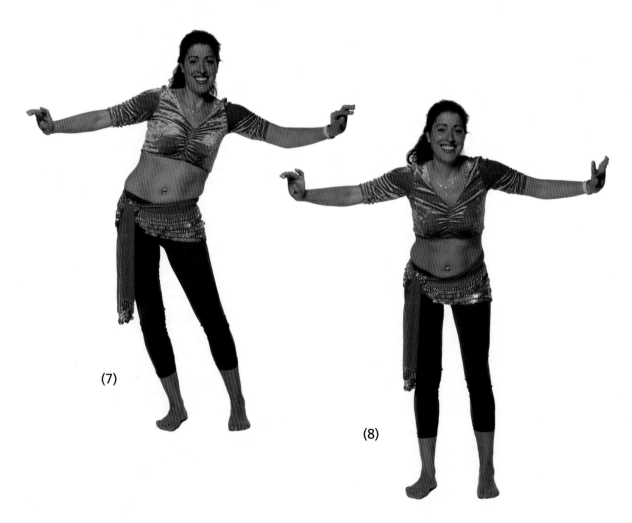

(7)

(8)

HIP CIRCLES VARIATION

You can also focus separately on each hip by doing half-circles on each side of your body. Begin by moving your pelvis forward (10). Then circle your hip backward, using your hip to draw a semicircle or half-moon shape over your right leg (7). You can then perform the same motion moving from back (8) to front (7). This exercise will allow you to train

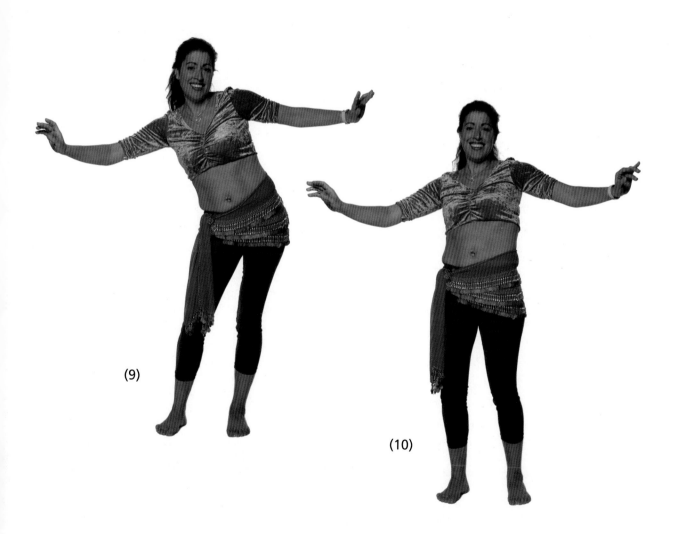

(9)

(10)

each side of your body intensively and strengthen any weak muscles. By performing hip half-circles, you may be able to feel the movement more easily and ensure that when you are doing your full hip circles, you work all of your abdominal area. Begin by performing these movements ten times on each side.

MANY-SIDED HIP BOWS

For the hip bows, picture yourself tracing a figure 8 on the wall behind you. The movement sequence goes like this.

For the hip bow to the right, press the right hip forward as you lift the heel and transition your weight onto the ball of the right foot. The left foot remains on the ground. Now move your chest to the left and let your weight shift to the left foot. The right foot flattens onto the ground.

To complete the bow, press the left hip forward, lifting the heel and taking your weight on the ball of your left foot. The right foot stays on the ground. Move your chest to the right and let your weight shift to the right foot. This completes one cycle of the movement.

Once you become familiar with the movement sequence for the hip bow, concentrate on making fluid transitions from one side to the other. Perform this exercise ten times. The hip bow can be varied in many ways—feel free to innovate!

THE "LYING" 8

With your hips you can trace the outlines of a figure 8 on the ground below you. Imagine a large 8 on the ground; position yourself in the center of the figure. Your weight rests evenly on both feet.

To begin the movement, press the left hip forward. The pelvis is now positioned on a diagonal line, the right hip pressing to the back. Shift your weight to your right foot and push the right hip a little further back. Make a half-circle to the front with the right hip—this will move the left hip backward, with the pelvis again positioned on a diagonal line. Move the weight to the left foot and push your left hip back a little. Now make a half-circle to the front with the left hip.

Continue moving from right to left and back again. The movements are fluid. The feet remain flat on the ground during this exercise. Perform this exercise ten times on each side.

This movement can also be done by taking your hips to the back and doing a half-circle from the front to the back.

FURTHER VARIATIONS OF HIP CIRCLES

Performing small circles using one of your legs as a pivot point is another hip circle variation. You can also move your entire body, turning in a complete circle while simultaneously circling your hips. If you are circling to your left, your left foot will be your stationary pivot point.

To perform this move, circle your hips as you step to the left with your right leg, turning your body with each step to complete a circle. This movement may be difficult at first as you try to sync up your circling and stepping. Creating a rhythm will make your steps look elegant. Circle four to five times to each side.

HIP LIFTS

For the hip lift, begin with your weight resting on the left foot; your right foot rests on the ball of the foot (11). Swing the right hip up as you rise on your right foot (12). The upward swing of the hips is strong. When the hip swings up, the foot on that same side turns inward slightly as if you were extinguishing a cigarette with the ball of that foot. The upper body remains steady.

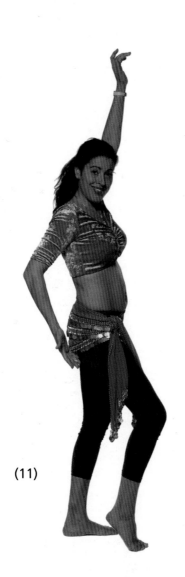

(11)

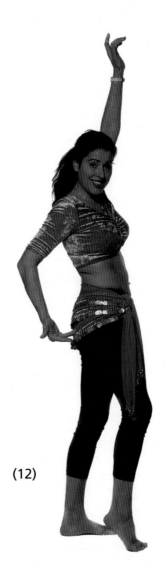

(12)

Practice this movement ten times on each side. Make sure that you are really popping your hip upward.

HIP SWING STEP

The weight rests on the right foot. Do a hip swing with the left hip and, at the same time, take a step forward with your left foot. Then do the

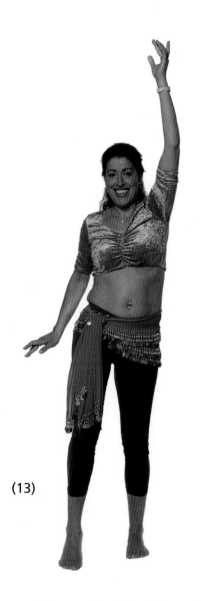

(13)

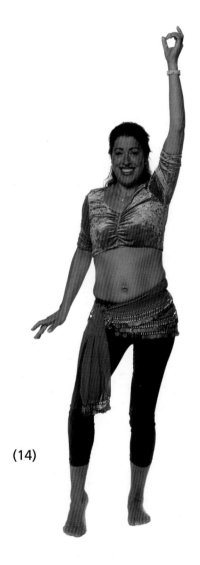

(14)

same thing on the right side—swing the right hip up while stepping forward with the right foot (13). Try to take a few steps in a row. Then
change to the left leg and develop the steps from the swing of the right
hip. You can vary these steps by practicing them while switching sides
(14). Try to take ten to fifteen steps.

HIP SWING CIRCLE

With the hip swing you can rotate around your own axis. When your left hip swings up, extend the movement by turning to the center in the swing. The right foot stays on the ground and turns as the left hip turns.

Practice four big swings or eight to ten small swings as you turn around your own axis.

PLAYING WITH THE HIP DROP

Opposite to the hip swing, the hip drop is a downward movement of the hip.

Rest your weight on the left foot. Using the ball of the right foot, press the right hip up and then let it fall. A traditional pantomime exercise teaches this sequence well. Imagine yourself approaching a bar stool. You lift your hip to reach the height of the stool and then let your hip drop as you sit on the stool.

Now switch to your right foot and let the left hip drop.

Play with this movement. Do two hip drops in a row, then move the weight to the other foot and do two hip drops. Change sides again. Do this exercise ten times with each hip.

THE HIP DROP STEP

Although many of these steps you have learned may seem to be stationary, most belly dancers move vibrantly around the room during the course of their routines. The hip drop step will allow you to stay in the mood of the dance while also changing your physical location.

To perform the hip drop step, begin with your weight on your right leg, in the position for performing a left hip drop. Drop your left hip, transferring your weight to your left foot, and then take a small step forward with your right foot. With your weight on your left foot, drop your right hip (transferring your weight to your right leg) and step forward with your left foot. Then perform a left hip drop and step forward with your right foot. Repeating this step, you can move as quickly or as slowly around the room as you would like.

When you are first learning this move try to make ten to fifteen fluid and connected steps. To challenge yourself, vary the music that you dance to and see how quickly or slowly you can perform this movement.

THE HIP DROP CIRCLE

In the same way that you performed a full-body turn while hip circling, you can perform a full-body turn while doing hip drop steps. Begin with your weight on your left leg. This leg will be your pivot point. Perform a right hip drop, then take a small step forward with your right foot. Transfer your weight back to your left foot and perform another right hip drop. You are pivoting around your left leg, so your weight will rest on that side throughout this movement.

After each right hip drop, take a small, quick step forward and perform another hip drop, turning around your stationary left leg until you have completed a full circle. Then switch and circle around your right leg.

This movement may seem complicated, but once you get into a rhythm it will become easier. Focus on each movement; many beginning dancers worry too much about circling and forget to drop their hip with emphasis. When you have mastered the basic movement, challenge yourself by varying the speed at which you perform this movement.

Moving the Chest

Isolating the movements of the rib cage might require even more practice than for the pelvic area and hips. While we're used to feeling the hips articulate when we walk, the rib cage generally stays quieter in everyday movement. The rib cage can produce isolated movements, however, and it is beautiful to see the range of motion available once we loosen this area of the body.

For a basic exercise to warm the muscles and move the bones of the chest cavity, stretch your arms sideways to a horizontal position without raising your shoulders. Move your rib cage to the right, picturing yourself reaching for a rope on your right side. Return to the center. Now reach to the left by moving your rib cage that way as you stretch your arm to grab an imaginary rope.

Keep your breath steady and deep as you perform this movement. You can support this movement by taking deep breaths at the beginning to lift the rib cage. Remain quiet in the hips and do not bend at the waist as you reach. Reach five times to each side.

LIFTING THE RIB CAGE

Take a deep breath and lift the rib cage (15). Picture a string in the middle of the chest pulling the chest cavity forward. Let the chest drop again and relax (16). Repeat this exercise five to eight times.

You can vary the raising of the chest by pulling the chest up on the right and left sides and dropping it back into the middle. Try making a V with the chest: up to the right, back to the center, up to the left, back to the center. Make your V starting on each side so that you develop equal abilities on both sides.

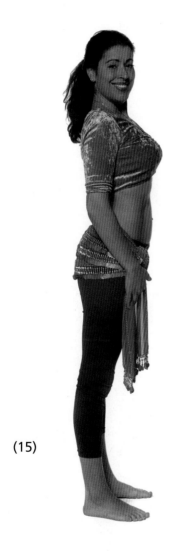

(15)

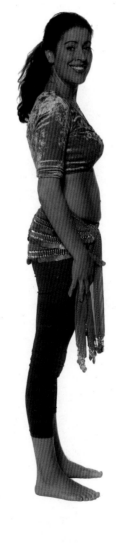

(16)

CHEST CIRCLES

Picture a square. Outline it with your chest by trying to reach all four corners from the inside. This increases the range of motion for the chest. Once you feel comfortable outlining the square, move toward making

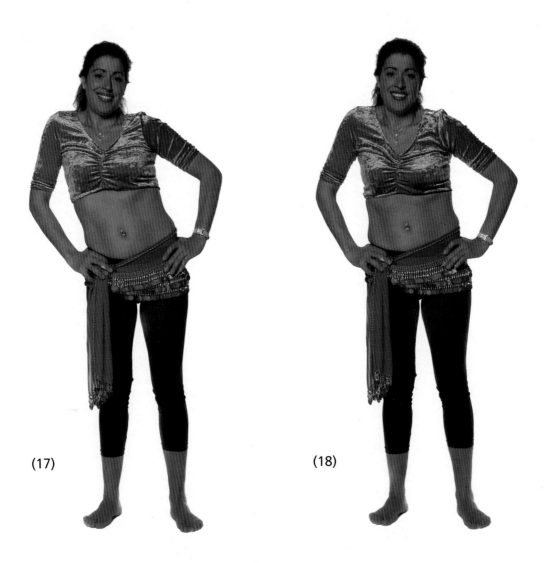

(17)

(18)

fluid circles with the rib cage (17–20). Circle five times to the right, then five times to the left.

If you have difficulty isolating the chest from the pelvis, it may help to stand with your back against the wall. Press your pelvis firmly against the wall to keep it steady.

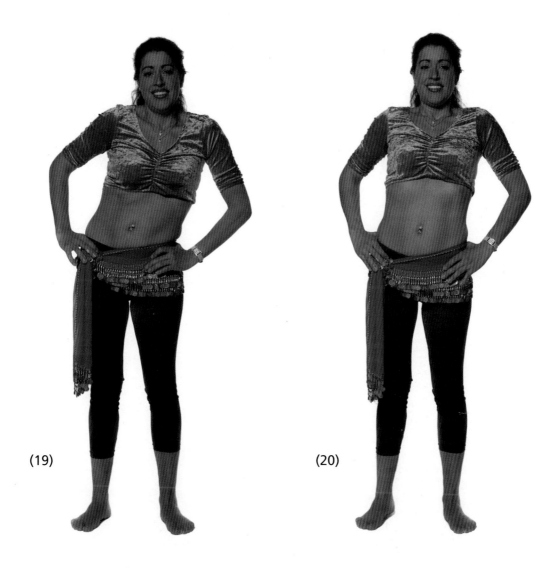

(19)   (20)

THE CHEST WAVE

Start in the basic position. Place your thumbs on your hip bones (21). Keep control of your shoulders during this exercise.

Inhale as you picture your chest being pulled upward by a string (22). Exhale and drop the chest back (23). This movement slightly adjusts the shoulder blades outward. The movement comes from the chest cavity; the shoulders do not move.

Return to the starting position and keep breathing steadily. Repeat the exercise four to five times.

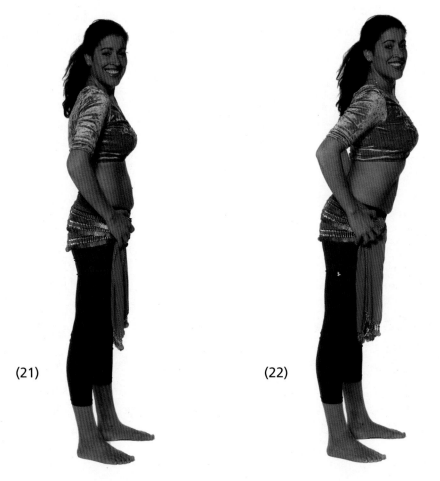

(21)   (22)

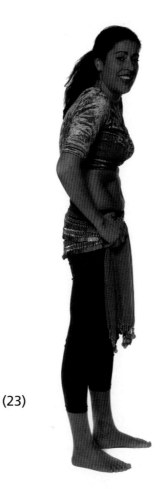

(23)

FIGURE 8 WAVES

When you are practiced in isolating your rib cage, you can begin practicing moving your chest in figure 8s. Make sure your movements originate from the chest muscles and not the shoulders. As with all the chest exercises, your shoulders should not move as you make these figure 8s.

Imagine a large figure 8 on the ground beneath you; position yourself in the center of the figure. Your weight rests evenly on both feet. Hold the shoulders steady. Beginning at the center of your imaginary figure 8, use your chest cavity to trace the loops on the floor. Really use your imagination with the exercise; it may help to make an actual 8 on the floor with tape so that you can be sure to make nice full loops with your chest. Remember, you need to hold your shoulders still, so it may help to do this exercise with a partner who can watch for shoulder movement and perhaps lightly hold your shoulders so you can practice isolating your rib cage. Do this exercise five to eight times.

SHOULDER SHIMMIES

During shoulder shimmies the chest remains steady. Picture yourself kicking a ball away from you first with one shoulder (24) and then with the other (25). Once you feel comfortable doing these movements slowly,

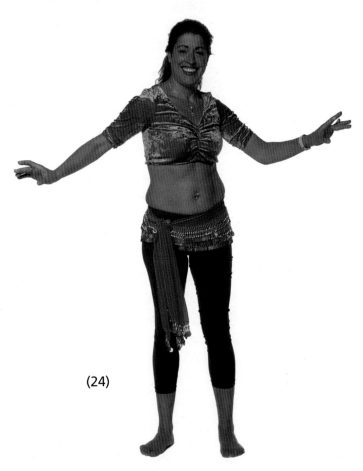

(24)

you can increase the pace to pick up with a quicker rhythm.

The following exercise will facilitate learning shoulder shimmies. Begin by sitting on the floor with your legs straight. Put your arms at your sides. Shake your upper body while keeping your shoulders steady. In this position you will gain a feeling for the vibrations of the chest.

Once you feel comfortable that the movement is coming only from your chest, lift your arms to your sides while continuing the shaking movement. If you lose the rhythm, put your arms down to your side and begin again. In time you'll develop the ability to shimmy from the chest only.

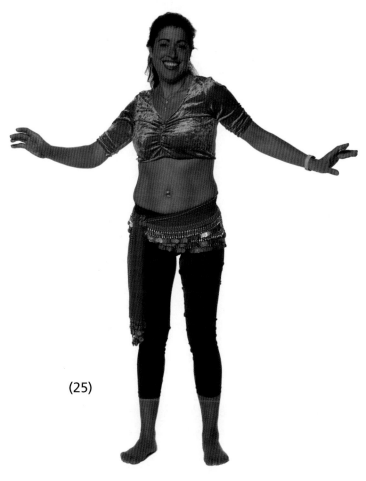

(25)

The Language of the Hands

In belly dance, hands are an important means of expression. Hand movements are also surprisingly difficult to learn. Beginning dancers tend to focus so much on the hips, chest, and other large body parts that they forget to work on holding their hands gracefully. Speaking through the movement of the hands adds a personal touch to the dance. The more flexible your hands are, the easier you can express certain emotions.

In most Mediterranean countries, as well as in Africa and Asia, hands are used with dramatic flourish in conversations to differentiate between different topics or underline the drama of a situation. In flamenco, in Thai dance, and in Indian temple dances, the movements of the hands are considered a special skill of dancers. A beautiful posture of the hands adds elegance and ease to the dance.

The following exercises support the development of grace in the hands and fingers. You may want to practice dancing in front of a mirror, watching how you hold your hands. Make sure that your hands look graceful and fluid as you move the rest of your body.

STRENGTHENING THE WRISTS

Position your hands at chest level without raising your shoulders. Make your hands into fists and then spread your fingers; simultaneously lift your elbows until they point sideways away from your body. Take a few breaths, then lower the elbows to your side. Shake out your hands and wrists.

This exercise strengthens the fingers and the muscles of the lower arms. Do it as often as you wish.

Here is another good exercise for strengthening the arms. Stretch your arms sideways away from your body. Make your hands into fists. Circle your fists five times to the outside and then five times to the inside. Now imagine small figure 8s on the ground below your wrists. Try to trace those small figure 8s with your wrists.

Shake out the arms and wrists. Repeat the exercise with hands spread, keeping the hand relaxed and the fingers loose. The wrist leads the movement; the hand follows.

PREPARATION FOR THE HAND WAVES

Position your hands at chest level without raising your shoulders. The hands are touching from the fingertips through the wrists (26). Keeping the thumbs and wrists in contact, gently press the fingertips together, creating a hollow space between the palms (27). From this position spread the

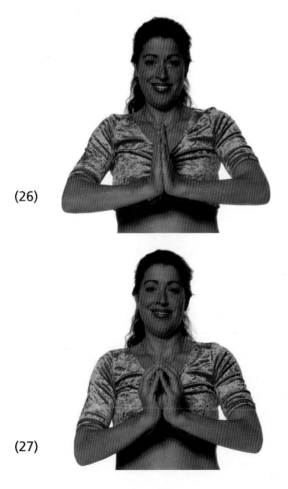

(26)

(27)

fingers, keeping the fingertips connected. The hands now look like claws. Maintain the tension for a moment, then slowly stretch the fingers upward to the starting position.

After practicing this preliminary hand exercise a few times, bring your hands into the claw position and then move your arms and hands in a large, sweeping motion. Imagine that you are swimming through deep water. You will want to do this exercise in front of a mirror because it is important that you develop graceful arm movements along with your dance. Repeat five times. After each repetition, briefly shake out your fingers and wrists.

SPREADING AND CLAWING THE FINGERS

Put your arms to your sides. Spread your fingers so that the tension reaches into the fingertips. Cup your palms and pull your fingers together into claws.

Alternate between spreading and clawing. Repeat ten times. Finish by shaking out the wrists.

THE PINCER GRIP

The pincer grip is a nice hand position for the dance. All fingers are slightly spread. The thumb and middle finger form slightly opened scissors. The middle finger is fully extended (28).

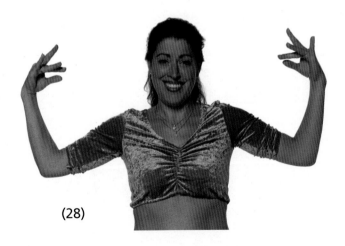

(28)

You can also open and close the "scissors" a few times—touching the tips of the thumb with the middle finger—to strengthen the fingers further. You can practice the pincer grip with each possible combination of thumb and finger: thumb/index finger, thumb/middle finger, thumb/ring finger, and thumb/little finger.

FIGURE 8 WITH THE HANDS

The hands are spread upward and held at the height of the buttocks. The fingers are pointing backward. Bring your wrists inward, in front of the navel, having them almost touch. Then flip your hands so that they are open, the palms pointing upward and the fingertips pointing toward one another. Bring your hands backward, past your hips, to the sides of your buttocks. Turn the fingers in a small circle from inside to outside until they point backward, as they did in the starting position.

You can also do this exercise at your sides, above your hips. Turn your upper body to the right while keeping your pelvis forward and make three figure 8s with your hand above the right hip. Then turn your upper body to the left and make three figure 8s above the left hip with your hand.

The Arms as Graceful Companions

Like your hands, it is very important that your arms also move gracefully as you dance. Think of your arms as water, flowing and flexing with ease. Arm movements help you to connect to your audience because by reaching out you can draw a person into the dance and into your performance.

Since arm movements are so essential for connecting with your audience, you should practice using arm movements in your dance. You may want to try dancing in front of a mirror while paying special attention to how you move your arms.

RELAXED SHOULDERS

Bring your hands together in front of your chest, your lower arms parallel to the floor and the elbows pointing outward. Keep the shoulders relaxed and away from the ears.

Tense your arms and press your palms against one another. Keep the tension up for a moment while continuing to breathe normally, then release the tension. Repeat five times.

ARMS IN HIP POSITION

Place your hands next to your hips, palms facing upward and thumbs pointing outward. You can use this hand position to accentuate the hip swing. You can also vary the hand position by turning the thumbs inward and facing the palms downward.

Turn your hands four to five times up and down by rotating your wrists. This arm position can accompany many dance moves—hip circles, hip lifts, and hip drops. You can also use this hand position while turning.

ARMS FOR GRACEFUL FRAMING

One hand is next to the hip, the palm pointing up. The other arm is slightly bent and held high with the palm above the head, the hand framing the head. Make sure that your hands curve gracefully as a part of your arm.

Try switching arm positions rapidly and "pop" your hips. When you pop your hip, you move it upward forcefully, like a champagne cork popping out of a bottle. Experiment with this arm position—it's great for emphasizing hip and pelvic movements.

WELCOMING ARMS

In this position the hands are held at the hips, palms open and fingertips pointing forward. Move your palms toward one another, having them meet in front of the pelvis about a foot from the navel. Your hands will be held in front of your pelvis, palms together. The upper body moves slightly forward.

Now open your hands, exposing your palms as though you were receiving a precious gift. Move your arms forward in front of you; at the farthest part of your reach, circle your arms back toward your body, leaving your palms open. When you reach the furthest point of the circle your upper body opens completely and your chest will thrust out. At the end, the palms are back at hip level.

This movement of the welcoming arms combines well with small hip circles. Practice this movement four to five times.

FOR BEAUTIFUL ARMS

For this exercise, imagine your hand as a paintbrush with which you're painting a wall in big strokes.

Stretch both arms in front of your body at chest level. Now move the right arm upward, above the head, while moving the left arm downward in a parallel motion (29). As soon as the right hand is above the head, flip the hand up from the wrist so that the palm is now facing outward. As soon as the left hand is at the pubic bone level, flip the palm toward the body (30). You should pretend that your arms are paint brushes and you are gracefully painting the space in front of you as you move each arm up and down. Practice moving your arms fluidly as you change from side to side (31). Your movements should not be jerky. Do this exercise ten times.

SNAKE ARMS

This movement comes from the shoulder. Practice it first with one arm before trying it with both arms.

Bend your right arm slightly at your side, the elbow pointing upward. Picture your elbow loosely hanging from a string, as if you were a puppet (32). Push your right shoulder forward and back a few times. Now lift the shoulder up and press it down a few times, always keeping the arm passive.

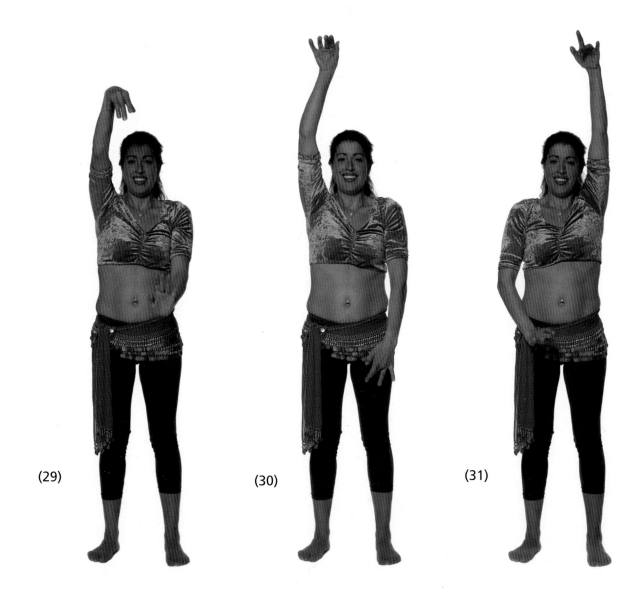

(29)   (30)   (31)

Now do the same movements with your left shoulder. The movement comes from your shoulder and should allow your arm to move like a snake twisting along the ground. Remember to keep your arm loose and fluid. Do this movement at least five times on each side.

Now lift the right arm above your head, with the palm pointing inward, toward your body. As soon as the hand is over the head, flip the hand up from your wrist (33). Now move the arm back down to hip

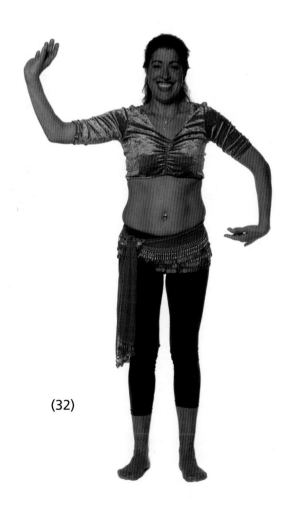

(32)

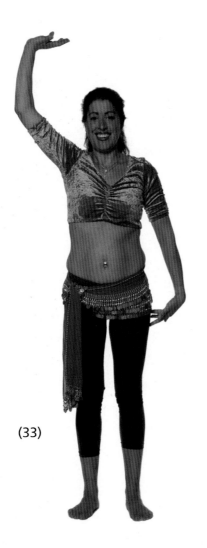

(33)

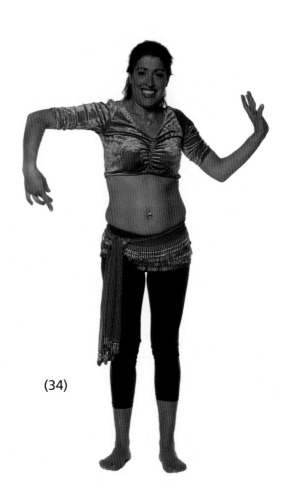

(34)

height, keeping the palm facing outward. The palm is folded inward and once again points toward the body (34).

Practice this movement five times on the right side. Switch and repeat with the left arm. When the arm is lifting, the movement comes from the shoulder. Nonetheless, take care to press your shoulder down as you lift your arm; the shoulders should not creep up toward the ears. This will cause the movement to lose its elegance.

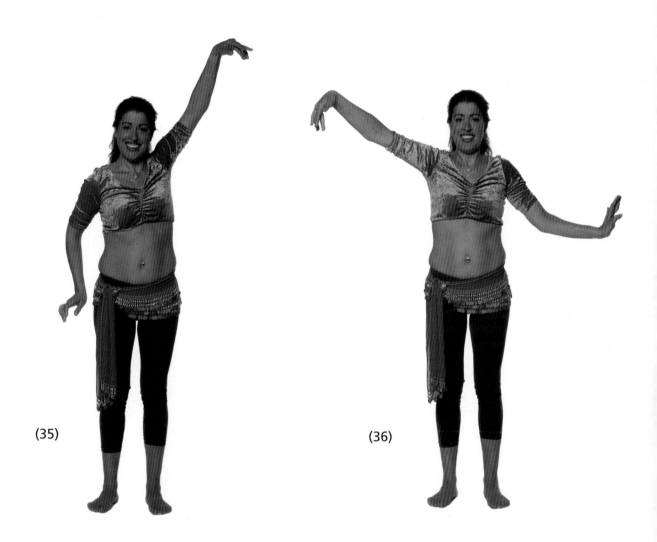

(35)

(36)

When you feel comfortable with this exercise, you can move both arms together. This means that while the right arm is moving down the left arm is moving up, over your head. Then you flip the left wrist up and begin moving the left arm down while the right arm moves upward (35).

Try moving both arms together ten times. You can also combine this movement with snake arms (36). However, this movement combination requires good motor planning (brain/body coordination).

FLYING ARMS

For this exercise, you will use your arms like wings.

Move your arms up and down on the sides of your body like a bird's wings. The movements should be easy and graceful. Begin by being slow and conscious of your movements, shaking your shoulders loose when you need to. Breathe regularly.

Do this exercise ten times.

HAND WAVES ENRICH THE ARM MOVEMENTS

You can add whimsy to your arm movements. Cross your arms at chest level. From your wrist, develop hand waves that continue into your fingertips. Open your arms outward, cross them again, and again begin the wave movement.

Put one hand to your temple and make small hand circles with the other hand. Picture yourself reaching for an apple with the hand. Move the hand from the head level in small circles down along your hips. At hip level, change the roles of the hands.

RELAXATION FOR THE ARMS

After working with these exercises it's good to relax the arms.

Lift the right arm up above the head and extend the left arm to your side (37). Picture both of your hands

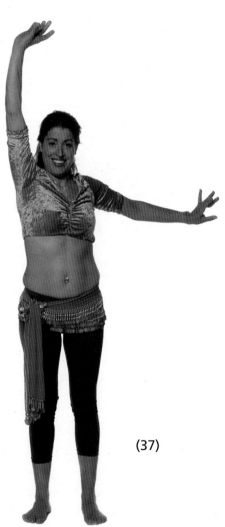

(37)

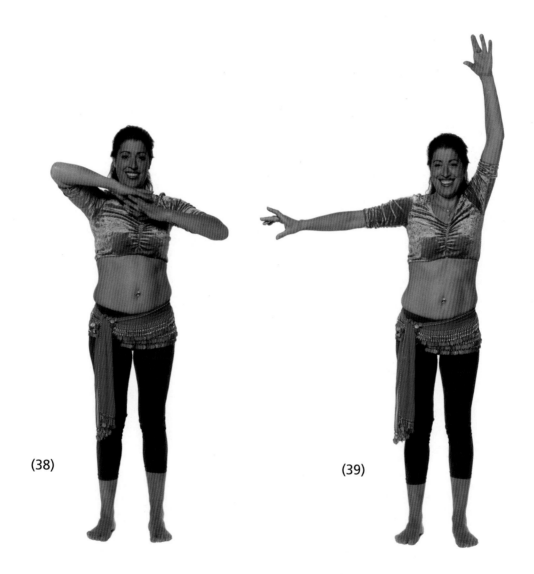

(38)

(39)

absorbing energy. Now move both arms toward one another. The hands meet at neck level and the palms move inward (38). Turn your palms outward and now stretch the left arm up and the right arm to the side (39). Repeat five to eight times.

This exercise strengthens the coordination of the arms.

Enticing Head Movements

Practice this exercise in front of a mirror. The movement comes from the lateral muscles of the neck, which we usually do not use and thus first have to discover.

Put your right hand to your right cheek. Press your cheek against your palm, keeping your head horizontal. Release your neck muscles and return your head back into its starting position. Repeat five times on the right side.

Now go to the left side. Put your left hand to your left cheek. Press your head against your left palm, tense, and relax.

When you've made good contact with your neck muscles and they feel enlivened and ready to "fire," fold your hands under your chin and move your head left and right using your hands. This enticing movement is especially well-suited for a dance with a veil.

Loosen your neck muscles by expressing small yes's and no's with your head. Move the head forward as though you wanted to avoid a touch to the back of your neck. Move back into the starting position and then move the head back, creating a double chin. Repeat five times.

Combine these forward and back movements with the sideways head sliding to create head circling. The head remains horizontal and circles around an imaginary axis.

Both head movements can be combined with the Turkish arm position (40 and 41). Keeping your shoulders down, take both arms above the head. Connect wrists and palms above the head to make a frame. Within this frame you can let your head circle or slide. The arms and the upper body remain steady. When the head moves to the right the eyes can turn left and vice versa.

This enticing movement originally hails from Indian dance.

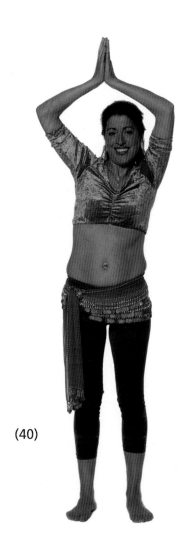

(40)

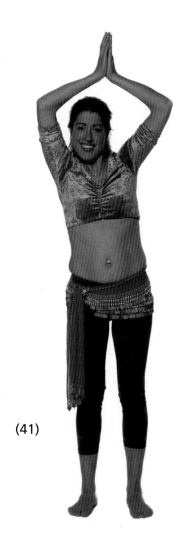

(41)

Shimmies

Even though shimmies are normally performed by more advanced dancers, most women would like to learn how to shimmy when they first begin dancing. The memory of having a dancer perform shimmies entices many women. As an aide, you should sling a cloth, preferably one with coins (a coin belt) around your hips. This helps you feel your hips more strongly.

When practicing shimmies, interrupt the exercise and loosen your body as soon as you feel as though you are cramping. Don't forget to breathe to avoid getting stitches in your side. It is helpful to learn shimmies in front of the mirror. The more you are able to let your body go, the easier it will be to learn these vibratory movements. Feel the powerful energy moving through your body. Release your power into the air around you by moving your hips.

Shimmies are well suited for dancing to drum rhythms.

FROM HIP SWINGS TO THE SHIMMY

Begin in the basic position. Tense your upper body while relaxing your pelvis and buttocks. The feet remain firmly on the ground (42). Begin with hip swings, moving your hips backward and forward. Increase the pace of the swinging motion. The faster you go, the smaller the swinging becomes until your hips eventually begin to vibrate.

SHIMMY WHILE SHIFTING YOUR WEIGHT

Start in the basic position. Shift your weight to your right foot. Begin with the shimmy and shift your weight to your left foot while your hip is vibrating. Move your weight back and forth between the two sides.

Try to make this movement as fluid as possible. Don't forget to breathe so as to avoid getting stitches in your side.

SHIMMY WHILE WALKING

As you move your weight to your right foot during a shimmy, try taking a step forward with your left foot without stopping the vibration. Shift your weight to your left foot and take a step with your right foot. Walking during shimmies requires good coordination and a lot of practice. Keep trying. Don't get frustrated if it takes you a long time to learn this move.

Another movement is to try walking backward or in circles. Don't for-

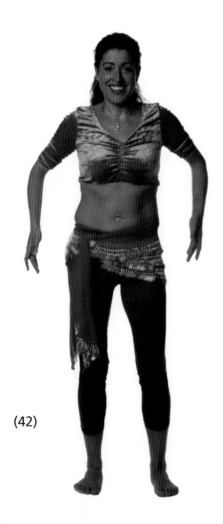

(42)

get to breathe. You can make level changes by rising on the balls of your feet for some steps and walking on flat feet for other steps.

SHIMMY FROM THE HIP SWINGS

Start in the basic position but bend a little deeper into your knees. Alternate between pushing the left and the right hip upward to the point where the knees are fully extended. Keep your feet flat on the ground. Increase the pace until these hip swings become a shimmy.

Relaxing Vibrations

This exercise is preparation for the shimmies. It relaxes the lumbar vertebrae and the calf muscles. It is especially soothing for pain in the legs or back caused by prolonged standing.

Lie on your back and bend your knees, keeping your feet flat on the floor. The feet are parallel to one another and facing forward. The angle of the legs should be such that the feet have no problem keeping contact with the ground and are at least one hand-length away from the buttocks. The knees are slightly opened.

Breathe calmly deep into your pelvis. Slowly begin to open your legs until the distance between your knees is approximately 12 to 16 inches, depending on the length of your legs. Now move the knees back toward each other until they're pointing straight upward again. The knees do not touch. Now open your legs again. The slow and conscious movement causes a slight tension in the leg muscles. You should notice this tension; if you don't, it might be that you are moving your legs too fast. If the exercise is done slowly, it will create a vibration within the leg muscles that will continue into the pelvis.

At first it will take ten to twenty repetitions or so to elicit these vibrations, but the vibrations will come more rapidly once you are familiar with this exercise. The exercise can also be easily done on the couch at night, for example while reading a book. Continue for as long as is comfortable, usually between five and thirty minutes.

THE SHAKING SHIMMY

The shaking shimmy is performed mainly by advanced dancers. During the shaking shimmy the vibration comes from all leg muscles. The strong contraction of the muscles leads to a moment where the legs start shaking. Advanced dancers are better able to isolate their hips. For example, they can vibrate their hips while doing circles with their upper bodies.

Fundamental Dance Steps

Even though they perform a lot of isolated movements, belly dancers are also able to move around the room. Remember, the dance can be performed to entertain others and to worship at the temple, where dancers would want to move around so that others could see the movements. Learning to circulate around the room, therefore, is an important skill for a dancer.

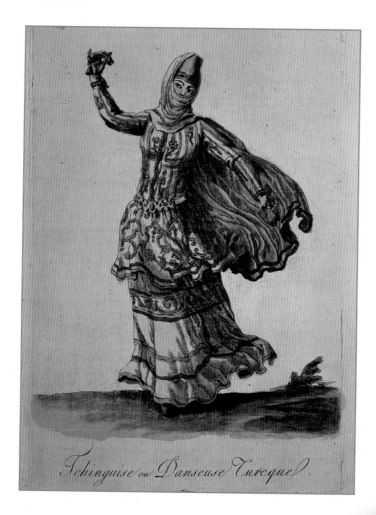

Tschinguise ou Danseuse Turque (Turkish Dancer), from Costumes civils actuels, Paris, 1788.

Incorporate these steps into your choreography so that you can dance around the room while also performing the isolated movements. Many beginning dancers find moving around the room while dancing to be difficult at first. Keep practicing. Group classes can be particularly helpful for learning how to move about a dance floor because the group moves together and participants can provide feedback to one other.

THE ARABIC BASIC STEP

Start in the basic position with knees extended (but not locked). Take a step forward with your left foot. Raise your right foot and place it down again in the same spot. Now raise the left foot and return it to the same spot.

Take a step forward with the right foot. Lift the left foot, then place it down in the same spot. Now lift the right foot and place it down in the same spot.

Take a step forward with the left foot and begin the sequence again: raise your right foot and place it down in the same spot; raise the left foot and return it to the same spot; take a step forward with the right foot.

This step can be combined with a number of different chest movements. The step can also be danced on the balls of the feet. You can take small steps and combine the steps with a hip swing.

THE SIMPLE ROTATION

Rotations accentuate a dancer's grace.

To practice rotations, begin in the basic position. Lift your arms to your sides. Turn once around your axis toward the right. Try to make the rotation in three or four steps, or even in a single step. Before you turn, fix on a steady point at eye level. While turning, look at this point for as long as possible. At the last moment turn your head and immediately "spot" this point again. This is the way dancers make successive turns without getting dizzy.

Saber Dance

Saber dancing can be learned in belly dancing classes. The tradition of dancing with sabers builds on the theme of women capable of defending themselves. Think of the tale of the smart Scheherazade from the "Arabian Nights," where the brave slave Morgiane twice saves the life of Ali Baba. The second time she performs a belly dance after dinner while carrying a dagger in her belt. The cook was beating the drum for the dance, and although the robber is annoyed because he had wanted to use the opportunity after dinner to kill his host, the rules of etiquette do not allow him to refuse the dance. At the end of the dance, Morgiane drives the dagger into the heart of the robber masquerading as a merchant and thus saves the life of her master. As a reward, she is given her freedom and the son of Ali Baba as her husband.

Among the four caliphs of Islam there were still courageous women who led armies and fought side by side with the men. The women of the Hamzar tribe, for example, rode on horseback and fought with their sabers in the manner of the Amazons. They defended their land and their religion against Christians and other tribes. Greek historians describe ritual dances of the Amazons that they conducted in full fighting gear to honor their mother goddess Kybele (another name for Artemis). The Amazons were believed to be the daughters of the war god Ares and, according to the historian Herodotus, were a female nomad tribe from the area between Skythia and Pontos. The great temple of Artemis at Ephesus, one of the Seven Wonders of the World, was supposedly built in an area controlled by Amazons.

FORWARD–BACKWARD STEP

Begin this step with the weight resting on the left leg. Take a step forward with the right foot, then briefly lift the left foot. Place the left foot back on the floor and shift the weight to that foot.

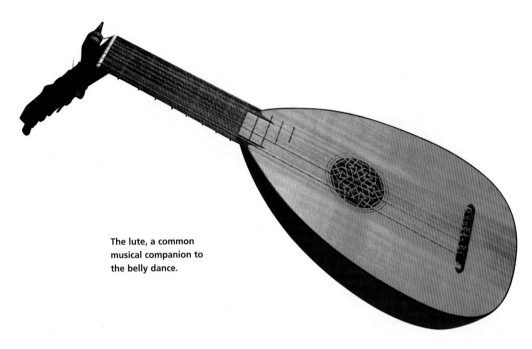

The lute, a common musical companion to the belly dance.

connect your mind and body and let your identity shine through. A class may help you think of new things and inspire you. Working with other women and experiencing their energies can be a helpful way to work on your own dance practice.

Challenge yourself every day to work on new combinations and to express your body in different ways. Remember to practice movements to both the right and the left so that you develop strength on both sides of your body. You might consider beginning every practice session with a visualization or by writing a journal entry so that you really think about what energies are inspiring you for that day. Seeing your belly dancing as exercise for your mind and your body will help you to make time for it in your busy life. Having a journal will allow you to reflect back over the years on what has inspired you to dance, and practicing visualizations can help you transition from a stressful day into a calming belly dance session. Ultimately you dance for yourself, so experiment to see which routines work for you.

Rhythms for Belly Dance

You can belly dance to many different types of music. Some people use belly dance moves when dancing to Western music while others prefer more traditional rhythms.

Cymbals and Castanets

The word *cymbal* is derived from Cybele, the Phrygian mother goddess from Anatolia. The original cymbals were bigger than those used today. Miniatures from Ottoman times show dancers with sticks of wood. They accentuated the musical rhythms in ways similar to the way in which cymbals are used. These sticks were called *kas* or *kasat* in Arabic, the precursor to the word *castanets*.

In playing with cymbals the dancer adopts the rhythm of the drum. There are special cymbal courses for beginners and experts. It takes some patience and practice to connect the dance moves, the musical rhythms and cymbal playing. But those who discover the charm of the cymbals would not want to dance without them.

Cymbals or castanets can help you to feel the beat of the music more forcefully. Furthermore, some musicians may want to improvise their own beats on top of the music to add creativity and personality to the dance. Practicing with cymbals may also help you to develop stronger hand and arm muscles and also develop extra grace in your arm movements.

If you would like to try cymbals, experiment to see which kinds work best for you. You should be comfortable using them. Cymbals should add to your dance, not distract from it.

Again, this may be a good time to think of your goddess archetype and what cymbals she might choose. Which instruments speak to you as you dance? We encourage you to go to a music store and play around with the selection. With some patience, you will find the instrument that will work in your dance practice.

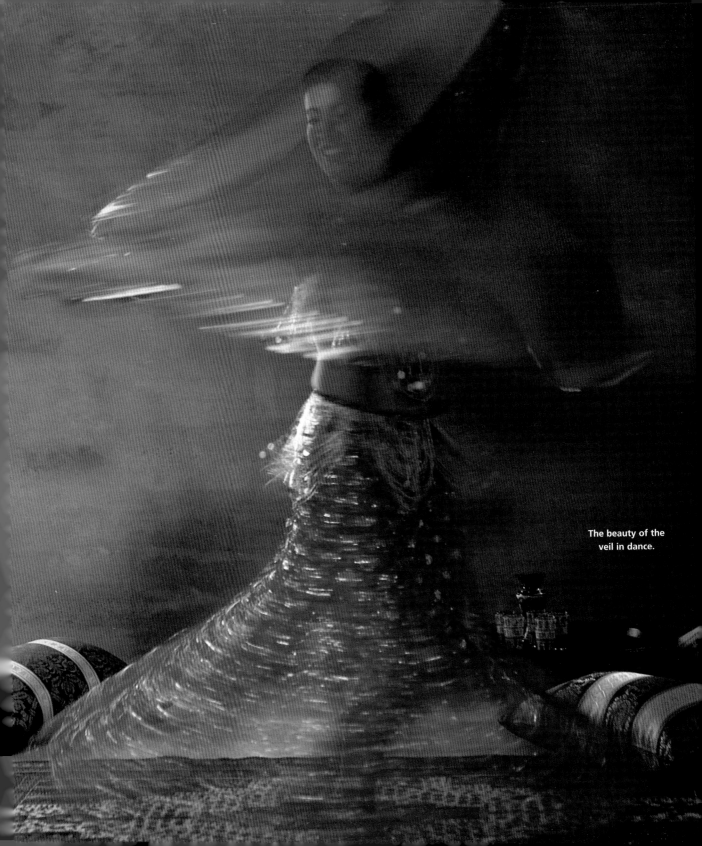

The beauty of the veil in dance.

Here is some information to help you choose appropriate music for your dance practice.

SOLO: THE TAQSIM

A *taqsim* is a solo musical piece. In Arabic music a taqsim is often a flute solo while in Turkish or Armenian music a taqsim is usually a clarinet solo. The taqsim is usually slow and hypnotic. It is good for arm movements, soft pelvic circles, upper body waves, and light turns.

DRAMA: THE BALADI

The dramatic rhythm of the baladi is easily recognizable through the strong double beat of the drum at the beginning of each phrase. It is suitable for strong dancing. You can accentuate the double beat through isolated movements of the pelvis or upper body.

The baladi is good for hip swinging, be it stationary, while walking, or during a turn. The deeper sound of the drum, produced by striking the middle of the drum, is called "dum." The lighter sound, "tak," is produced by hitting the edges of the drum.

The basic rhythm of the 4/4 baladi is "dum dum tak tak dum tak tak," pause, and repeat.

SENSUAL AND EXOTIC: THE CIFTETELLI

This slow but strong rhythm is easily recognized by the three strong beats at the end of each unit. In Arabic music, drum accents are varied from one unit to another. In Turkish music the beat is slower and heavier. The instruments interpret each unit in the same way. The rhythm has a very sensual and exotic mood.

The *ciftetelli* is good for arm movements, hip circles, slow walking, and turns. The beat of the 8/4 ciftetelli is "dum-take-tak-tak-dum-dum-tak" ("take" refers to a quick after-beat on the left).

Clothing That Enhances the Dance

Your costume will be an essential part of your dance practice. It is very important to pick a costume that fits well, that makes you feel comfortable, and that gives you support in movement. Going to a belly dance class or costume shop and speaking with a costuming expert can help you to find the perfect outfit for your dance practice.

There is a wide variety of costume choices. Some women dress in loose pants or skirts with a bra-like top to accentuate the belly; others choose to cover the abdomen with sheer fabric. You can tie scarves or coin belts around your hips for emphasis; some women like to emphasize their arms with bangles or arm bands.

Look around at other dancers to see what costumes you like and try on different things while dancing to get a better idea of what will work for you. Again, journaling or visualizing your goddess archetype may help you to decide on a comfortable and appropriate costume. Although finding a flashy costume may be fun at first, it is important to consider how the costume works within your dance practice.

In addition to the fit of your costume, the color will also be very important because colors express different moods and part of the body (see the box on the chakras on the next page). The wonderful colors of the Middle East and Asia entrance the senses. The film "Monsoon Wedding" by the Mira Nai is a stunning example of the wealth of colors at an Indian wedding. Those who have traveled through the Middle East or India know the colorful array of spices on the market: yellow saffron, red chilies, brown cumin, red-brown cinnamon, olive laurel leafs.

Red, black, white, and yellow were the first colors to be given names by mankind. In Africa, colors are important not only for their symbolism but also as medicine. The Mesopotamians decorated their temples with the colors that corresponded to their heavenly gods. The Egyptians not only painted their buildings and sculptures but also themselves. Red colors were

Understanding the Chakras

Chakra teachings relate the colors of the rainbow—the spectral colors—to centers of spiritual strength in the human body. The word *chakra,* from Sanskrit, means "wheel" or "circle." According to the chakra teachings, the energies of the chakras surround the body like an aura and represent the spiritual strength of the body or the soul.

Being a key manner of aura manifestation, in chakra teachings colors are viewed in relation to a person's spiritual condition. An animated and vivacious person prefers strong colors such as red; the person's aura would be associated with that color as well. Conversely, wearing the color red would give energy to someone who is feeling depressed or downtrodden. The colors in a room can also have an effect on a person's moods.

The chakra centers are located along the spine. These energy centers need to be open and unobstructed for the human body to function at maximum efficiency. Color therapy may help you to open any chakras that feel weak or blocked.

- First chakra: Otherwise known as the base or root chakra, this chakra is located at the tip of the tailbone, equidistant between the anus and genitals, and includes the feet and legs. The color associated with this chakra is red. The internal organs most affected by this chakra are the uterus and ovaries and the prostate and testicles.

- Second chakra: This chakra is located between the pubis and the navel along the front of the spine. The color associated with this chakra is orange. Orange is considered to be a healing color for depressions and psychoses. The internal organs most affected by this chakra are the intestines.

- Third chakra: The solar plexus chakra is located three centimeters above the navel at the front of the spine. The color associated with this chakra is yellow or gold. Yellow stands for the sun and intellect;

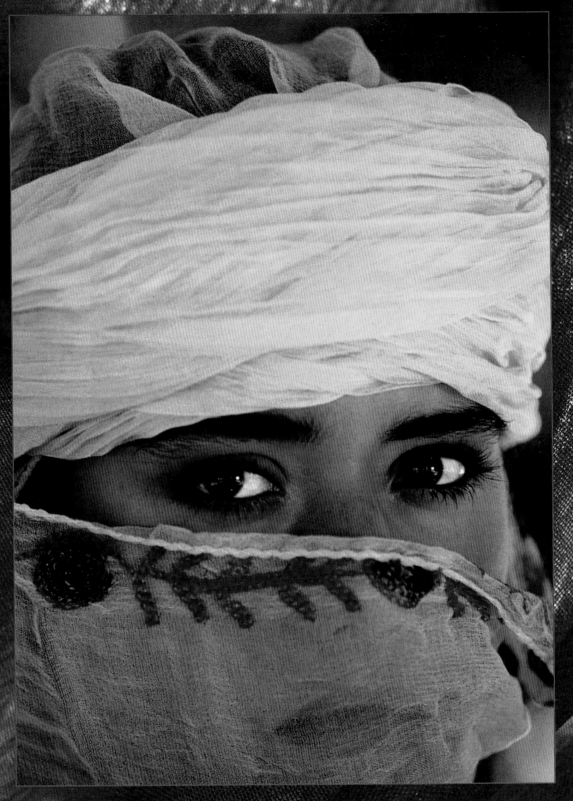

The veil adds an element of mystery to the dance.

their hair as an offering. This practice could be seen at the temples of Artemis, where girls who were about to be married left a lock of hair along with their childhood toys at the temple.

During Mohammed's lifetime the veil was still considered a fashion accessory for wealthy women. To protect their chastity, Mohammed counseled women "not to display their charms more than what is visible by necessity, and cover their chests with veils and reveal their charms in front of nobody but their husbands and fathers." Mohammed was speaking about the breasts, not the face. Parallel with the demise of the Omaijaden dynasty in Damascus, which was an aristocratic society in which many women had wealth and education, conservative theological views gained currency. It was under the reign of the Abbasids at the court of Baghdad, especially under the narrow-minded caliph al-Kadir, that women were banned from public life and confined to the harem. From then on, the complete covering of the body with a veil was demanded.

Along with the harems, the Abbasids adopted the customs of Persian royalty and eventually lost Arabic customs. In contrast to the free Arabic women, Persian women were oppressed, although in modern times the wearing of the veil has spread across the Middle East. The veil became a duty especially for women in the cities. In rural areas and in the desert, women retained their original freedom. Female Bedouins didn't (and in some cases still do not) wear a veil. They looked after the tribe's day-to-day existence and a veil would have disrupted their work. In some tribes, men too wore veils to protect themselves from the evil eye. To many observers, the female Bedouin embodied the self-sufficiency and the dignity of the free Arab woman.

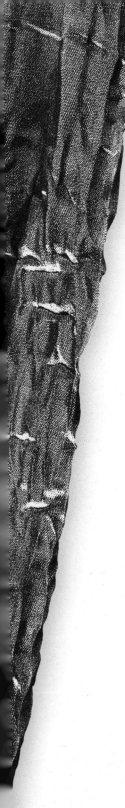

Belly Dance:
An Emotional, Physical, and Spiritual Exercise

As we have seen in our study of the dance, belly dance allows women to express their sensuality and strength, adds grace and balance to the body's carriage, and makes the muscles more limber. Belly dance can help you to connect to your inner spiritual health and express that spirituality through movements. As you practice the dance, remember to allow energy to flow through your body.

Beginning with the strengthening and stretching exercises discussed in the last chapter and progressing to the fluid dance moves may seem like an endless journey—which, in a sense, it is. With dedicated practice, you will develop the muscles, strength, and skills to dance beautifully. However, you will also find that belly dance is a skill that can constantly be improved and the exercises and movements presented in this book will help both advanced and beginning dancers make their dances more meaningful and graceful.

In the next chapter, we will consider how to bring your other senses to your dance practice. As you improve your dancing, you may want to experiment with foods, scents, and cosmetics that allow you to more fully experience the world of belly dance. By integrating the external world with your internal experience, you can turn belly dancing into a ritual that you can share with your friends and family.

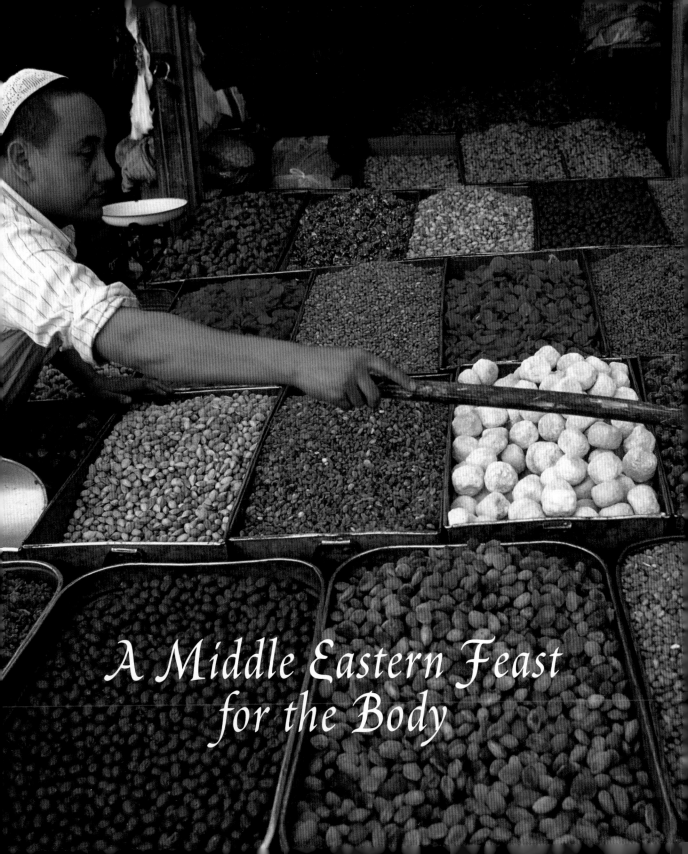

A Middle Eastern Feast
for the Body

*W*eekend and weeklong workshops are the best way to quickly but fully enter the world of belly dance. All across the United States and Europe, reputable and experienced teachers lead seminars that cover belly dance basics in depth, providing the beginner with an immersion into the feelings of physical and spiritual well-being, relaxation, beauty, sensuality, and enjoyment that belly dance can bring. It is easier to learn dance moves in this kind of relaxed but directed atmosphere, and oftentimes new friendships take root in such a setting. As well, most women have an easier time learning belly dance in a group. If you can avail yourself of such an opportunity, this is a great way to take your belly dance study to the next level.

There are other elements of Middle Eastern culture that many women find themselves drawn to once they begin dancing. We've already discussed the urge toward color and beautiful fabrics that overtakes many women once they begin dancing. Middle Eastern music, which accompanies the dance, sometimes becomes a woman's preferred choice in sound. Middle Eastern scents and foods are two other domains of the senses that women who belly dance often find themselves drawn to.

Diving into Exotic Scents

The olfactory sense plays a significant role in our emotional well-being. The sense of smell acts mostly at the level of the subconscious; the olfactory nerves directly connect to the most primitive part of the brain, known as the

A MIDDLE EASTERN FEAST FOR THE BODY

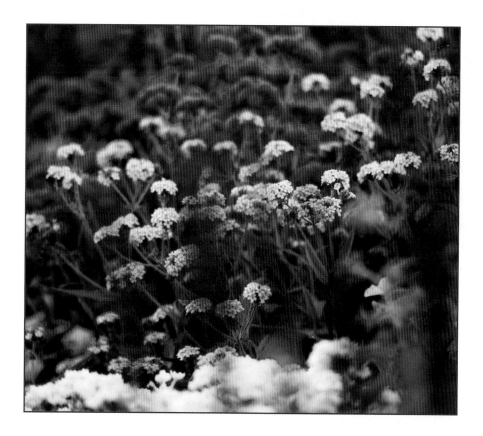

limbic system or the rhinencephalon ("smell brain"). Smell is the first sense that nature gave to life—long before sight or sound or even touch. If you want to immerse yourself in the life elixir that belly dance can be, certain aromas can help transport you.

Many perfumes today have Middle Eastern scent components, each of which is made up of between 150 and 200 individual ingredients. Often they are essential oils of flowers, petals, fruits, and herbs. Essences extracted from roots, onions, mushrooms, and bark also play an important role.

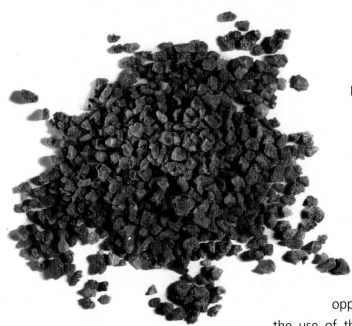

Perfumes with a Middle Eastern flavor used to contain natural animal ingredients such as musk, which was harvested from the sex gland of the male musk deer. Since the Asian musk deer is an endangered population, many people today oppose on political grounds the use of this substance in perfume making. Luckily, however, there are excellent synthetic musks that agree with most skin types, providing an alternative and allowing the heady scent to continue to be used by many. The same goes for ambergris, a substance that can be harvested from the intestines of the sperm whale. This scent is also frequently found in Middle Eastern perfumes, but here too the ban on whale hunting has resulted in the development of synthetic alternatives.

Woodsy scents derived from various tree juices and resins also play an important role in Middle Eastern perfumes. Frankincense is obtained from a tree that grows in the Arabian desert and on the Somali coast of Africa. Myrrh is a resin obtained from a shrub also found in Arabia and Somaliland. In addition to their wide use in perfume making, the ancient Egyptians used both substances for embalming their dead and for mummification.

The scent ingredients in perfumes are classified as either top notes, middle notes, or base notes.

Top notes are the boldest scent in a perfume blend. They give the first impression of the blend but do not last long. Top notes are mostly derived from flowers, fruits, and leaves. They constitute approximately 20 percent of a perfume blend.

Middle notes give body to a perfume. They are warm and mellow. Middle notes constitute the majority of a perfume blend.

Base notes deepen a blend and increase the perfume's lasting effects. Base notes constitute 10 to 20 percent of a perfume blend.

Making your own scent combinations can personalize a scent to you. We have included a few perfume recipes that you might want to experiment with. Or you can look for some of these ingredients in a commercially blended scent.

Pinette

Scent group: flowery, jasmine

4 drops amber oriental
3 drops wood classic
10 drops jasmine
6 drops rose
6 drops musk
15 drops cosmetic basic water

Midsummer Night Wind

Scent group: oriental spice

5 drops rose
3 drops amber oriental
25 drops wood classic
20 drops jasmine
10 drops lily of the valley
5 drops musk
3 drops ylang-ylang
18 drops cosmetic basic water

Aphrodite

Scent group: flowery amber

10 drops amber oriental
3 drops animal
10 drops wood classic
20 drops jasmine
15 drops lily of the valley
10 drops rose
5 drops orange oil
8 drops vanillin

Oriental Garden

Scent group: oriental, aromatic, musk

2 drops amber oriental
14 drops wood class
30 drops jasmine
7 drops rose
4 drops musk
19 drops orange petals
20 drops cumarin

A MIDDLE EASTERN FEAST FOR THE BODY

Preparing Delicious Food:
A Middle Eastern Buffet

Certainly one of the most pleasurable aspects of exploring Middle Eastern culture is the cuisine. The cuisine encompasses the foods of southern Europe, northern Africa, and the countries that surround the Mediterranean. Abounding in fruits, grains, legumes, vegetables, lamb and chicken, nuts, and olive oil as well as pungent spices and roasted flavors and spices, Mediterranean food provides a healthy diet of great variety. Indeed, the diet of the Middle East is one of the healthiest in the world and has recently been gaining attention as beneficial to the heart and for long life.

If you would like to introduce your friends to the magic of the Middle East, why not invite them for a Middle Eastern buffet? Here we give you a few classic recipes from the Mediterranean cuisine that will help you begin your culinary journey. For additional resources on Middle Eastern cooking see *A Mediterranean Feast* by Clifford Wright, *Mediterranean Street Food* by Anissa Helou, and *The Slow Mediterranean Kitchen* by Paula Wolfert, among many other fine cookbooks available.

Sesame Oil—A Blessing for Our Health

Sesame has long been used in the cuisine and the healing practices of Mediterranean cultures. Eating one teaspoon of sesame oil every day is beneficial to the body. No other oil has as high a content of unsaturated fatty acids. From a medical perspective, sesame oil supports circulation; the high lecithin content strengthens the nerves.

Sesame oil applied externally as a massage oil is good for the skin and hair. In his writings, Socrates made frequent mention of the healing powers of sesame.

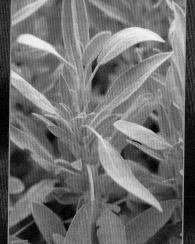
Bulgur, couscous, and millet are three of the grain staples used in Mediterranean cooking. Chickpeas (garbanzo beans) and lentils are some of the most popular legumes; they lend protein to nonmeat dishes.

Bulgur is wheat that has been steamed and then dried and cracked into pieces. This process reduces the starch content present in the wheat and thus makes it easier to digest. Bulgur contains all vitamins and minerals of whole-wheat grains and is very easy and quick to prepare. Bulgur is the main ingredient in tabouli.

A MIDDLE EASTERN FEAST FOR THE BODY

Couscous is the fine-grained variation of bulgur. Couscous is popular especially in Tunisia, Morocco, and Algeria. Bulgur and couscous are both good for a quick yet wholesome dish. Most children love couscous.

Millet is a mineral-rich grain that has been grown since prehistoric times. Its mineral content is especially good for strengthening skin, hair, and nails. Millet is easily digestible and helps support the healing of kidney and bladder infections.

Chickpeas are pureed with sesame tahini, olive oil, garlic, and lemon juice to make hummus, a popular Middle Eastern spread. Because of their high protein and starch content, meals with chickpeas are both filling and high in energy. Chickpeas take a while to cook. If you are short on time you can use canned chickpeas, available in health food stores and specialty groceries. Lentils are easily digestible and are high in proteins and carbohydrates. Lentil meals are thus especially frequent in countries where meat is not eaten for religious reasons. Lentils are a healthy alternative to meat.

The fresh orange color of carrot puree adds decoration to every buffet. Steam 500 grams carrots in water with some vegetable broth and puree the soft carrots in a blender. You can serve the carrots together with zucchini slices or steamed broccoli on a plate and decorate with herbs. You can refine the purees with olive oil or mascarpone.

An eggplant puree should be part of your Middle Eastern buffet. Cook one or two eggplants (depending on their size), puree them, and mix with olive oil, garlic, plenty of dill, pepper, salt, diced goat cheese, and chopped walnuts. Roasted eggplant rounds are also a wonderful addition to a *meze* (appetizer) plate. Round out your buffet with sliced peppers, tomatoes, carrots, and cucumbers, served with a yogurt dip. You can spice this yogurt with olive oil, lemon, finely chopped herbs (especially peppermint), or finely grated cucumber, as well as salt and pepper.

Finish off your buffet with a sweet dessert such as yogurt and fresh raspberries or halvah, a delicious sesame and honey candy. Mint tea is the beverage of choice to enjoy throughout your meal.

Bulgur

1 cup bulgur
2 cups water

Combine the bulgur and water and cook over medium heat for 10 minutes, or until the bulgur is soft.

You can also cook bulgur in vegetable or chicken broth. It tastes good when mixed with cold-pressed olive oil and steamed vegetables such as carrots, fennel, peppers, tomatoes, and zucchini.

Chickpeas

1 cup chickpeas (soaked
overnight)
4 cups water
pinch sea salt

Immerse chickpeas in a bowl of cold water. Shells and broken parts will float to the top and can be picked out by hand. Rinse and then cover the chickpeas with fresh water. Soak overnight.

Transfer the chickpeas and water to a large saucepan. Bring the chickpeas to a boil, then cover and simmer until the chickpeas are tender, approximately 90 minutes. The fresher the beans the quicker they will cook.

Use cooked chickpeas to make hummus. You can also mix them with grains, sprinkle on salads, or use in a stew with seasonal vegetables.

A MIDDLE EASTERN FEAST FOR THE BODY

Millet

1 cup millet
2½ cups water

Thoroughly wash the millet in hot water; this takes away its bitter taste.

In a medium saucepan, bring the water to a boil. You can add a teaspoon of vegetable broth or some sea salt to the water if you'd like. Add the millet, stir, and return to a boil. Cover and simmer for approximately 30 minutes.

Refine the millet with fresh spices such as basil or peppermint, tomato puree, or grated parmesan cheese. Or you may want to impart a sweet taste with ginger, anise, raisins, dates, and sesame.

Millet is very easy to digest. If you want to be good to your body, plan a "millet day" once a week on which you eat a bowl of millet for every meal. You can make it sweet or spicy according to your own taste. On this day, drink herbal teas, water at room temperature, and carrot juice (preferably freshly pressed).

Tabouli

1½ cups bulgur
2 cups boiling water
½ cup lemon juice
⅓ cup olive oil
3 cloves garlic, crushed
salt to taste
3 scallions, minced
3 plum tomatoes, diced
2 bunches parsley, minced
2 bunches peppermint, minced

Place the bulgur in a medium saucepan with a tight lid. Add the boiling water and let sit for 45 minutes.

In a blender or food processor, blend the lemon juice, olive oil, garlic, and salt until smooth.

When the bulgur is ready, drain well. You can line a strainer with cheesecloth, put the bulgur in the cheesecloth, and twist to take out all the excess water. Place the bulgur in a large bowl.

Add the lemon juice and olive oil dressing, scallions, tomatoes, parsley, and peppermint. Mix well and chill.

Serve tabouli on a bed of greens with olives and tomato slices. Tabouli is a wonderful accompaniment to humus pita pockets.

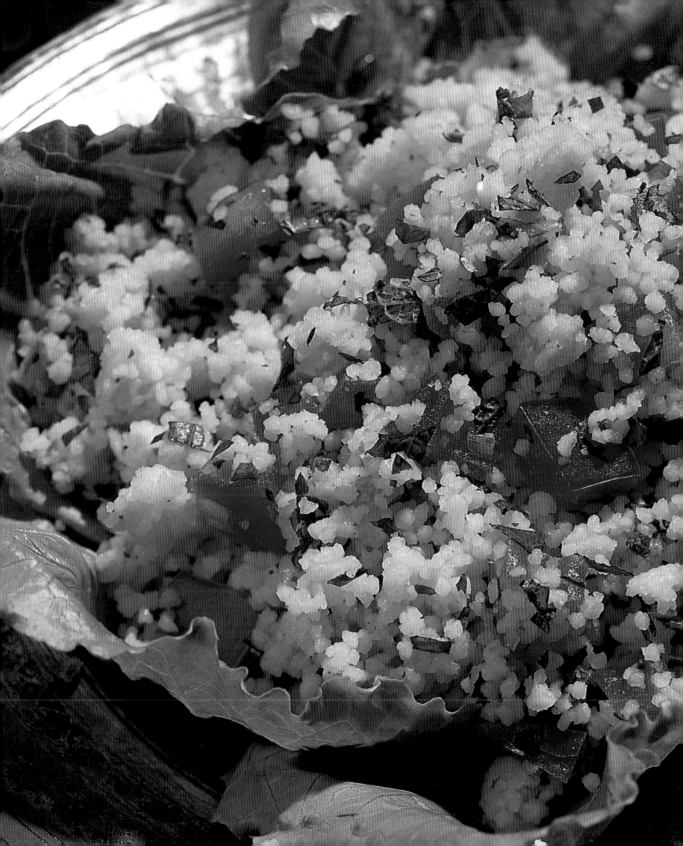

Hummus

2½ cups cooked chickpeas
2 cloves garlic, peeled
¼ cup tahini
2 tablespoons sesame oil
2 tablespoons lemon juice
1 tablespoon finely chopped parsley
salt and pepper to taste

Place the chickpeas and garlic in a food processor fitted with a steel blade. Puree until the chickpeas begin to break down.

Add the tahini, sesame oil, lemon juice, parsley, and salt and pepper. Puree until smooth.

Serve hummus on a bed of lettuce. Sprinkle with paprika. Or serve in pita bread with sprouts, tomatoes, goat cheese, and olives.

Praise for the Mint: Tea for the Buffet

With the buffet you can serve peppermint tea made from nana mint. Nana mint has less menthol than peppermint and is therefore more appealing than European mints to many people. Nana mint can be found online and in specialty tea shops.

The famous natural doctor and herbal healer Maurice Messegue writes: "The Arabs almost have a cult over the mint, and I freely agree with the praise. The lowest farmer will have a small peppermint bunch with him just like the most powerful emir." The nomads of the desert valued the antiseptic qualities of the mint.

Ancient peoples were very familiar with mint. They used its branches to make headgear for their ceremonies and used mint to treat snakebites and scorpion stings, colics, cough, nausea, all kinds of urinary problems, sexual dysfunction, and menstruation problems.

Messegue recommends the following brew once a day to support the treatment of impotence, orgasm problems, and to support sexual harmony: two pinches mint and one pinch savory for one cup of tea with boiling water.

A MIDDLE EASTERN FEAST FOR THE BODY

Chickpea Curry

1 tablespoon butter
3 cups cooked chickpeas
1 clove garlic, minced
1 teaspoon coriander
1 teaspoon turmeric
1 teaspoon cumin
one pinch each: ground cloves,
    cinnamon, nutmeg, ginger,
    salt
2 tablespoons fresh lemon or
    lime juice
4 tablespoons chopped parsley
sour cream

Melt the butter in a large skillet. Stir in the garlic, coriander, turmeric, cumin, cloves, cinnamon, nutmeg, ginger, and salt. Let the spices cook a moment, then add the chickpeas. Simmer the chickpeas in the spicy sauce for 15 minutes.

Sprinkle the lemon juice over the chickpeas and garnish with the parsley. Serve the chickpeas topped with a dallop of sour cream.

Salad-e-Sabzi

1 head of lettuce, roughly cut
1 small bunch Italian parsley
1 small bunch peppermint
1 small bunch chervil
1 bunch watercress
1 bunch radishes, sliced
1 small cucumber, diced
3 tomatoes, finely diced
2 scallions, finely chopped or
1 red onion, cut in half rings
½ cup olive oil
juice from 1 lemon or lime
herbs, finely chopped: basil,
    tarragon, marjoram,
    oregano
salt and pepper to taste.

Sabzi is the Persian word for greens and herbs.

Mix the greens with the radishes, cucumber, tomatoes, and onions.

Mix the olive oil with the lemon or lime juice, herbs, and salt and pepper. Toss the greens with the dressing and serve as a side dish.

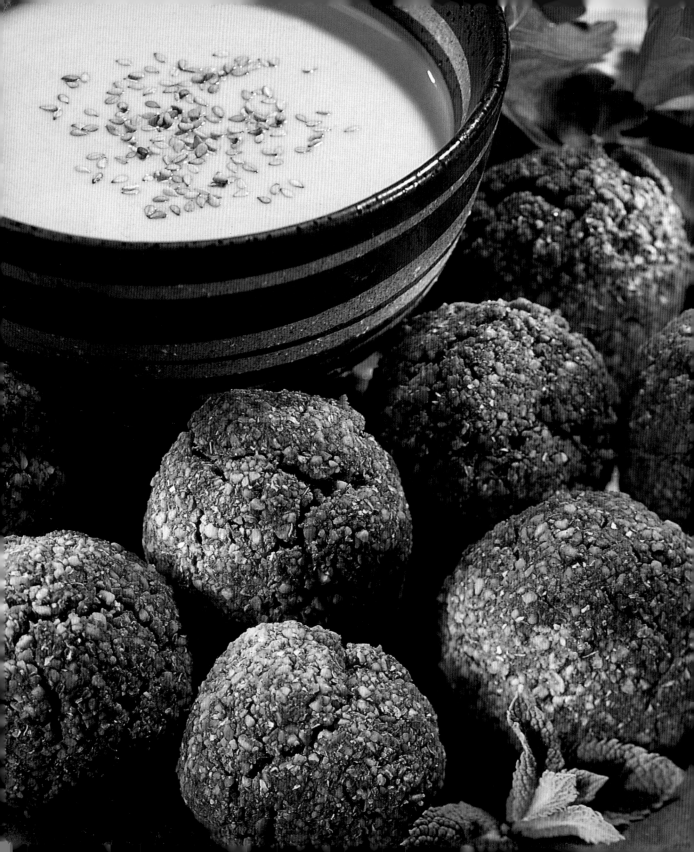

Falafel

1 cup raw chickpeas
$^1/_2$ teaspoon baking soda
1 cup boiling water
$^1/_4$ cup bulgur
1 or 2 cloves garlic, pressed
3 scallions, minced
$^1/_4$ cup sesame seeds
$^1/_2$ teaspoon ground cumin
$^1/_2$ teaspoon ground coriander
1 tablespoon finely chopped parsley

Cover the chickpeas with water, mix with the baking soda, and soak overnight.

Rinse the peas well. Place them in a food processor fitted with a steel blade and grind them finely.

Pour boiling water over the bulgur and let it stand for ten minutes, then drain and press out the excess water.

Mix all remaining ingredients and let the mixture rest for one hour.

Wet your hands and form flat balls out of the mixture, using two tablespoons for each ball. Let the falafel rest for another 30 minutes, then place them on a greased baking pan and bake them in the oven at 375° for 30 minutes.

Serve falafel with hummus, yogurt sauce, and pita bread. Ready-made falafel mix can be purchased at health food stores and specialty food markets.

A MIDDLE EASTERN FEAST FOR THE BODY

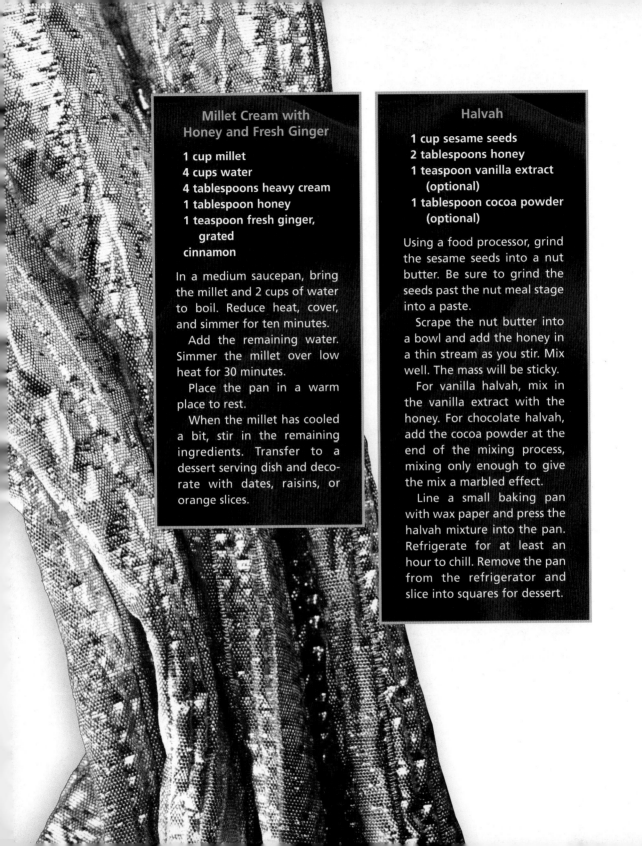

Millet Cream with Honey and Fresh Ginger

1 cup millet
4 cups water
4 tablespoons heavy cream
1 tablespoon honey
1 teaspoon fresh ginger, grated
cinnamon

In a medium saucepan, bring the millet and 2 cups of water to boil. Reduce heat, cover, and simmer for ten minutes.

Add the remaining water. Simmer the millet over low heat for 30 minutes.

Place the pan in a warm place to rest.

When the millet has cooled a bit, stir in the remaining ingredients. Transfer to a dessert serving dish and decorate with dates, raisins, or orange slices.

Halvah

1 cup sesame seeds
2 tablespoons honey
1 teaspoon vanilla extract (optional)
1 tablespoon cocoa powder (optional)

Using a food processor, grind the sesame seeds into a nut butter. Be sure to grind the seeds past the nut meal stage into a paste.

Scrape the nut butter into a bowl and add the honey in a thin stream as you stir. Mix well. The mass will be sticky.

For vanilla halvah, mix in the vanilla extract with the honey. For chocolate halvah, add the cocoa powder at the end of the mixing process, mixing only enough to give the mix a marbled effect.

Line a small baking pan with wax paper and press the halvah mixture into the pan. Refrigerate for at least an hour to chill. Remove the pan from the refrigerator and slice into squares for dessert.

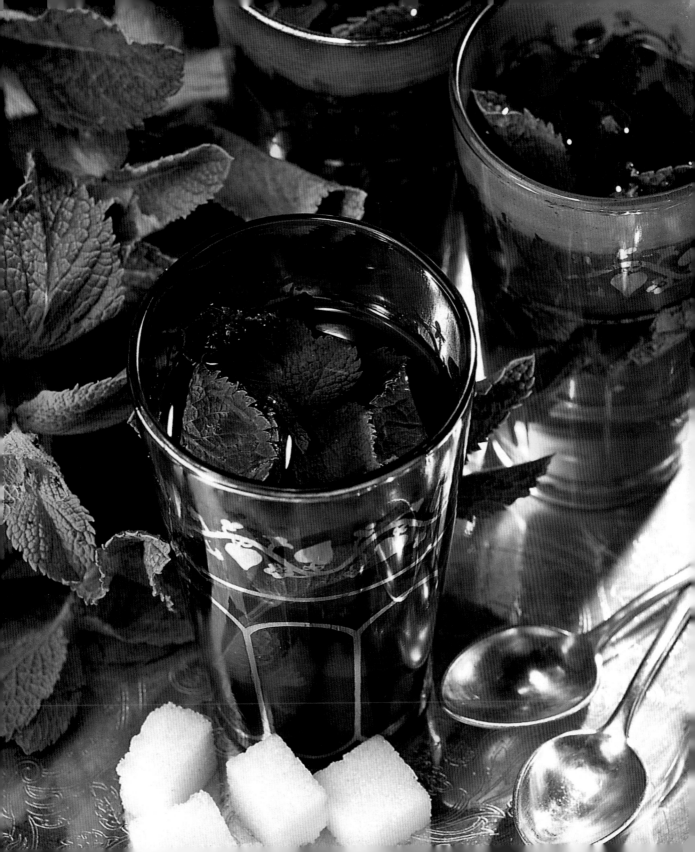

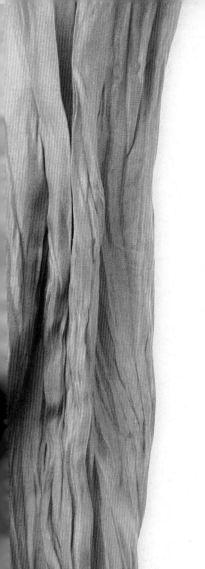

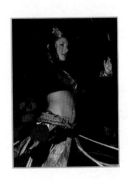

Resources

Teachers/Workshops

Gypsy Caravan

A modern tribal belly dance troupe founded in 1991 by artistic director Paulette Rees-Denis, Gypsy Caravan performs a modern eclectic style of belly dance that reflects ancient longings to celebrate community spirit and life mysteries. In addition to performing in Portland and throughout the northwest United States, Paulette and dancers teach around the country and in Europe. Performance videos, instructional videos, and cassettes of their original music are also available.

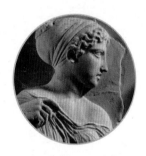

Caravan Studio/Gypsy Caravan

4050 NE Broadway

Portland, OR   97232

503.287.1794

www.gypsycaravan.us

Barika BellyDance

Barika Bellydance is a tribal fusion belly dance troupe based in Milwaukee. Barika, which means "to bloom" in Algerian, was founded by four women who wanted to share the wonderful connection and energy they found together through dance. Barika

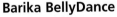

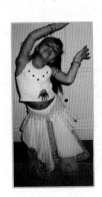

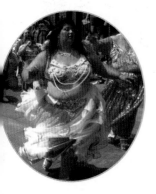

performs throughout the midwest. Barika also works within the community, teaching and mentoring young women through their ShimmyPower program. The goal of ShimmyPower is to promote positive self-image, good health practices, and empowerment through dance in a positive environment.

Barika Bellydance

Ami Hudson, director

414.562.9043

www.barikabellydance.com

FatChanceBellyDance

Since the creation of FatChanceBellyDance by Carolena Nericcio in 1987, the troupe has fascinated audiences worldwide with their exciting improvisational technique. Carolena has refined a montage of different elements into what has been coined American Tribal Style belly dance. The range of Carolena's comprehensive instructional videos, her interactive video consultation with remote students and teachers, as well as FCBD's commitment to out-of-town workshops have spread FCBD's American Tribal Style technique and philosophy around the globe. Online catalog.

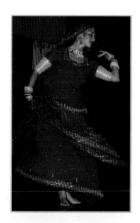

FatChanceBellyDance

PO Box 460594

San Francisco, CA 94146

415.431.4322

www.fcbd.com

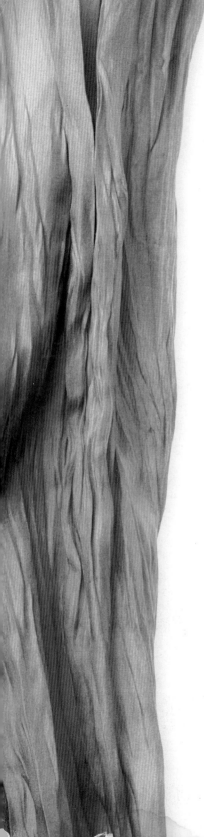

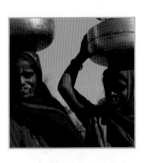

Videos

Suhalia Unveiled by Suhalia Salimpour

The Sensual Art of Belly Dance—Beyond Basic Dance
by Veena and Neena Bidasha

Belly Dancing: The Sensual Workout by Shamira

Egyptian Belly Dancing for Intermediates with Hilary
Thacker

Tribal Style Belly Dance, Vol. 1 with Kajira Djoumahna

Tribal Style Belly Dance, Vol. 2 with Kajira Djoumahna

21 Shimmies and 1001 Variations with Leyla Jouvana
and Roland

Belly Dance Spins and Turns with Marguerite

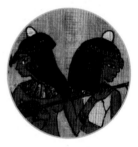

Music for Belly Dancing

Zaghareed by El Funoun

Music of the Fellahin, Music of the Ouled Nail, and
Music for Oriental Dance by Aisha Ali

Luxor to Isna by Musicians of the Nile

Belly Dance: A Gift from Cairo by Hamouda Ali

Best of Baladi and Saidi, Samya, and *Immortal Egypt*
by Hossam Ramzy

Melodic Musings by George Lammam

Khaliji by Souhail Kaspar and Naser Musa

The Magic Art of Belly Dancing by George Abdo

*Mystical Garden, Suleyman the Magnificent, Fire
Dance,* and *Whirling* by Omar Faruk Tekbilek

Passion Sources, a compilation by various artists

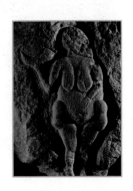

Suggested Reading

Tribal Bible: Exploring the Phenomenon That Is American Tribal Style Belly Dance by Kajira Djoumahna

Serpent of the Nile: Women and Dance in the Arab World by Wendy Buonaventura

Habibi Magazine: A Journal for Lovers of Middle Eastern Dance and Arts

Harem: The World Behind the Veil by Alev Lytle Croutier

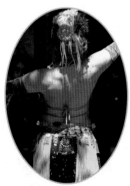

Online resources

The Gilded Serpent

An online resource in magazine format with articles ranging from historical research to up-to-the-minute news. Gilded Serpent's mission is to become Middle Eastern dance's journal of record.

www.gildedserpent.com

The International Academy of Middle Eastern Dance

An international association of dancers, instructors, choreographers, and musicians dedicated to promoting the art of belly dance through education about belly dancing history and artistry, performance and instructional videos, concerts and performance events, and the annual Awards of Belly dance recognizing outstanding artists and their contributions to the field. Suzy Evans, president.

www.bellydance.org

Books of Related Interest

Sacred Woman, Sacred Dance
Awakening Spirituality Through Movement and Ritual
by Iris J. Stewart

A Yoga of Indian Classical Dance
The Yogini's Mirror
by Roxanne Kamayani Gupta, Ph.D.

Offering from the Conscious Body
The Discipline of Authentic Movement
by Janet Adler

The Path of the Priestess
A Guidebook for Awakening the Divine Feminine
by Sharron Rose

Pilates on the Ball
A Comprehensive Book and DVD Workout
by Colleen Craig

Virgin Mother Crone
Myths and Mysteries of the Triple Goddess
by Donna Wilshire

Balancing Your Body
A Self-Help Approach to Rolfing Movement
by Mary Bond

Soul Talk
The New Spirituality of African American Women
by Akasha Gloria Hull

Inner Traditions • Bear & Company
P.O. Box 388
Rochester, VT 05767
1-800-246-8648
www.InnerTraditions.com
Or contact your local bookseller